The Art of Control

A Woman's Guide to Bladder Care

Copyright © 2015 by Leslie M. Parker.

All rights reserved. No part of this publication can be reproduced or transmitted in any form or by any means, electronic or mechanical, without permission in writing from the author or publisher.

Leslie M. Parker's

The Art of Control

A Woman's Guide to Bladder Care

Published 2015

Foreword

As a practicing physician in the field of Obstetrics and Gynecology, I have become accustomed to speaking with my patients about very sensitive issues. Issues that they likely have never spoken to anyone else about. Urinary incontinence as you can imagine and, maybe even relate to, tops the list.

As a matter of fact, if we don't ask our patients about their bladder health most women and men won't bring up their concerns due to a self-consciousness that equates to significant embarrassment on their part.

Lately many celebrities such as Kirstie Alley, Lisa Rinna and Whoopi Goldberg have taken to the stage and have gone in front of cameras to advocate for the millions of women who are suffering from urinary incontinence by becoming spokeswomen for incontinence pads. While I am grateful for the attention that their celebrity brings to this silent issue, I personally want more than a pad for my patients.

When I first met Leslie Parker, MPT, over six years ago, she came to my practice to introduce herself during a lunchtime meeting. At the time, we had a few physical therapists in the community that were working with our patients who suffered from incontinence. However, no one had ever come to us and proclaimed that they could help women start to get better within the first week of meeting with them.

Leslie definitely had my attention at that point. I left that meeting thinking, well, she seems nice enough and she seems to know what she is talking about but can she really deliver on what she promised? After all, most women have suffered for many, many years with incontinence before seeking help. How could they get better in just under a week?

Once a patient admits to suffering from urinary incontinence, whether it be stress incontinence, the type that causes leakage when you laugh, cough or sneeze, or urge incontinence, it's my job to counsel them on the options available to help them. In today's busy world often times I find my patients looking for that "magic pill" that will make everything better or asking for the surgery that their friend or relative had. I continue to be shocked when most of my patients have never even heard about the option of pelvic floor physical therapy to help them reach their goal of being dry.

I began to refer patients to Leslie and the feedback from my patients made me a believer in her straightforward, sensible approach to treating urinary incontinence and other bladder related issues. You will find the real truth about your bladder in her book. Leslie dispels many myths related to the bladder which will help women empower themselves to regain freedom from their pads. She has included a section on Tips of The Trade that answers common questions with workable solutions that she shares with her own office patients on a daily basis.

I am grateful that my patients can benefit from working directly with Leslie. Through this book Leslie now can reach out to the millions of men and women who suffer silently with bladder dysfunction. You won't find a "magic pill" reference or recommended surgical approach to treat your urinary symptoms in this book. Instead, you will learn to make lifestyle changes that are lasting. You'll learn techniques that will empower you to strengthen your pelvic floor on your own and most of all many of you will never need to buy another urinary incontinence pad again.

Dr. Colene Arnold
FACOG, Obstetrics and Gynecology
Garrison Women's Health Center
Dover, New Hampshire

What Others Are Saying ...

"I am delighted to be able to refer women with bladder issues to Leslie. Her compassion, knowledge, and skills combine to help women get results. Leslie's book is a great aid and resource for women and professionals to use for pelvic floor and bladder health."
—Susan M. Hollinger, APRN

"Over the last 20 years I have had the privilege of watching Leslie grow from a fledgling pelvic floor therapist into a master of pelvic muscle rehabilitation. Her limitations in this field are only set by her aspirations. I hope that Leslie will continue to share her practiced knowledge and wisdom to patients and clinicians alike in the coming years. I can't wait to see what she will do next."
—Earl Carlow, CEO, Current Medical Technologies, Inc., Lakeville, MA

"I found out about Leslie's practice after suffering with interstitial cystitis, constipation, pelvic pain, and levator spasms. In other words, my intestinal system and bladder issues had increased to a point of inability to travel, or even to function. Luckily, one of my doctor's told me to try to find a pelvic pain therapist. Leslie is one of few in my area with this type of knowledge and expertise. For the past two years, I have seen Leslie on and off. Her advice and her methods of physical therapy have helped me to vastly improve. Leslie is kind, gentle, and extremely knowledgeable. She WILL help anyone with improving their health because she is intuitive and honest about overall health, and specific problems related to the pelvic area. Leslie has connections to appropriate doctors, and she is highly respected. Do not hesitate to make an appointment."

—Karlene Dell'Ova, Durham, NH

"I have had the privilege of personally referring my patients with a variety of pelvic floor disorders to Leslie Parker, MPT. Uniformly the feedback that I receive regarding her approach to treating these disorders is fantastic. Women experience positive results much quicker than either they or I could ever imagine."

—Dr. Colene Arnold, Garrison Women's Health Center, Dover, NH

"Leslie Parker demystifies incontinence, bladder issues, and pelvic pain through easy-to-understand explanations and humor-filled candor. Her step-by-step resolutions to problems deemed "incurable" by so many physicians showcase her rarefied knowledge and give readers a new lease on life."

—Health Writer, Victoria Veilleux

"I found out about Leslie from my yoga instructor. I am so thankful. I had been dealing with hip pain, back pain, knee pain, and ankle pain for many months. In five minutes, Leslie recognized that my pelvis was out of alignment, and this turned out to be what was causing all of my symptoms. She taught my husband and me how to realign my pelvis. She wanted me to rely on her as little as possible. I have to say too, I really enjoyed working with Leslie. She is perceptive and direct and a go-getter. I am so appreciative of the healing help Leslie gave me."

—Susan Gross, York, Maine

"I am so very happy to have this opportunity to share what a great experience I have had working with Leslie. Most women I know don't want to talk about anything that is out of the norm "down there". You don't find urinary incontinence or pelvic floor issues at dinner parties or BBQs. Being able to ask questions and have them answered in a way that is easy to understand, with kindness and humor, made a whole lot of difference and sense in my everyday life!"

"We put together an action plan, I follow it, and all is well – simple, easy, DONE! Gone are the days running to the bathroom in a panic and not wanting to drink ANYTHING ... while I travel. Thank you!!!"

—EJW, Jamaica

"I rely on Leslie's expertise as a physical therapist and as an expert in pelvic floor dysfunction, disorders of the bladder and GI track. Her knowledge and skills are often an integral part of the treatment plan for many of my clients with bowel and bladder conditions. I am happy to refer my clients to Leslie and to work together to coordinate care for our mutual clients."

—Maria Larkin, MEd, RDN, LD, CLT of Better Gut Better Health, L.L.C

Dedications and Appreciations

This book is the product of many hours of thought, planning, writing, rewriting, and dedication. None of it would have been possible without the help of my very good friend Ruth Eurenius. She was my rock. Her unwavering advice and motivation is what kept me going, even when the going got tough. I am indebted to her for all her support and encouragement and I dedicate this book to her.

To my husband, Steven Parker, and our three sons, Max, Noel, and Rees: You are my world. Thank you for giving me the time and space to follow my dream. Your patience and support did not go unnoticed. I appreciate your confidence in me and love you all to the moon and back!

Thank you, too, to Hattie Stiles for the beautiful cover art and to Jen Kelly for the wonderful interior illustrations. They are fantastic!

"If you want something you've never had, you must do something you've never done."

—Oprah Winfrey

THE ART OF CONTROL
A WOMAN'S GUIDE TO BLADDER CARE
OUTLINE

Introduction	1
Chapter 1: Urine Trouble Now	3

   The Problem
   The Progression
   The Solution

Chapter 2: Test-Taking 101	7

   Urinary Incontinence Impact Questionnaire Pre-Program
      Blank & Sample
      Directions
   Input & Output Diary Pre-Program
      Blank & Sample
      Directions

Chapter 3: Muscle Power	15

   General Bladder Function
   Resting vs. Contracting Bladder
   Meet Judy
   Warning

Chapter 4: One Drop Is A Leak	19

   Detailed Bladder Function
   Normal vs. Not Normal
   Bladder Shrinkage
   Nighttime Waking
   Warning

Chapter 5: You Irritate Me   22
   Bladder Irritation Consequences
   Bladder Fatigue
   Ferocious Four
   Invisible Irritants

Chapter 6: The Truth About Poop   28
   Bowel Function
   The Bowel's Relationship To The Bladder
   The Bowel's Role in Urinary Frequency
   The Bowel's Role in Urinary Urgency
   The Bowel's Role in Urinary Leakage
   The Bowel's Role in Organ Prolapse

Chapter 7: The Constipation Revelation   35
   Definition of Constipation
   Causes
   Treatment

Chapter 8: It's About Time   41
   Key Components of Fluid Intake
      How Much to Drink
      What to Drink
      When to Drink
   Lucky Liquids
   Bladder's Rate of Fill

Chapter 9: Rush Hour   44
   Meet Mary
   Urgency Issues
   Autonomic Nervous System's Role
   Treatment

Chapter 10: Bigger Really Is Better   50
   Stretching The Bladder
   The Signal System
   Peeing 'Just In Case'
   Nighttime Fringe Benefits

Chapter 11: More Muscles That Matter   54
   Pelvic Floor Muscles
   Location
   Function
   Problems

Chapter 12: The Inside Workout   57
  Kegel
  Roll-In
  The Pelvic Brace

Chapter 13: What Goes In Must Come Out   66
  Judy's Urinary Incontinence Impact Questionnaire
  Judy's Input / Output Diary
  Analysis of Judy's Input / Output Diary
  Judy's Outcomes

Chapter 14: The Medication Fixation & Surgery Surge   75
  Medications
  Weaning Off Medications
  Surgery And Side Effects

Chapter 15: Do As I Say <u>And</u> As I Do   79
  Comprehensive Home Exercise Program
    Fluid Intake Schedule
    Urgency Program
    Fluid Output Schedule
    Exercise

Chapter 16: FAQs & Tricks of the Trade   83
  Questions
  Answers
  Tricks of the trade

Chapter 17: Diary of a Wimpy Bladder   94
  Judy's Outcomes
  Interpretation

Chapter 18: Test-Taking 102   97
  Judy's Urinary Incontinence Impact Questionnaire Pre-Program
  Judy's Urinary Incontinence Impact Questionnaire Post-Program

Resources For Incontinence   101

Glossary   103

For More Information   109

Introduction

At 22 years old, I had a Bachelor of Science degree in management information systems (computers) and no idea what I wanted to do with the rest of my life. I worked in the computer industry for several years but without fulfillment. I returned to school to begin a master's degree in accounting hoping this would excite me. After a year of courses, accounting was not interesting enough to hold my attention. I continued working, all the while wondering what I really wanted to do.

I met my husband, who worked for a large medical facility as a physician assistant specializing in pediatric medicine, in 1992. His work piqued my interest and, with his direction and support, I again decided to return to school. As they say, the third time's a charm. In 1994, I was accepted into the Master of Physical Therapy Program at Notre Dame College in Manchester, NH, where I met Patricia Wolfe.

Pat was a physical therapist who specialized in women's health issues. She was the head of the Rehabilitation Department at Portsmouth Regional Hospital, a large seacoast area hospital. Pat taught a women's health course during one of my semesters at Notre Dame College. She was fabulous. She exuded knowledge, confidence and passion in her teaching. It truly inspired me.

The day I met Pat was the day I finally knew what I wanted to do with the rest of my life. Here was a woman who, in one hour, was able to solidify my niche in PT. That was no small feat.

During my early practice as a physical therapist, I began to see more and more problems of incontinence in varying degrees. It was the problem women least wanted to talk about with their physicians. In fact, they never mentioned it unless their physicians asked. Unfortunately, most doctors did not ask. Unsurprisingly, most of the doctors who did ask were usually women.

These women needed guidance and support. To help them, I had to learn too. The process was trial and error with some methods more successful than others. This book is a result of all our early efforts.

Twenty years later, I am a physical therapist specializing in women's health issues, just like Pat. My program helped thousands of women, and by making a few simple changes it can change your life too. I still love to help women get their lives back. It is as simple as that. This is what I was meant to do!

Chapter 1
Urine Trouble Now

The Problem
The Progression
The Solution

The Problem

So, your bladder is not behaving. Why now? Why is today any different from yesterday? Your bladder always behaved before, but today it decided to act up. So what do you do now?

Too bad there isn't a Super Nanny for bladders that misbehave ... or is there? Well, stop the press because there is one now, and it is me! Just think of me as The Super Bladder Nanny. Ok, laugh if you must, but I find it quite catchy. After all, I have been called stranger things by previous patients and colleagues throughout my professional years, only with the nicest of intentions (I hope). One young woman who was ecstatic with her physical therapy outcomes lovingly mentioned that she referred to me as her PPT (i.e., Pee Physical Therapist) when she was with her closest of friends. How cute is that? I loved it and surely will never forget it.

I have also been referred to as The Bladder Queen, The Pee Pee Avenger, The Miracle Worker, The Wonder Pee Woman, and the Bladder Witch. I'm still not sure which one is my favorite, although I am partial to PPT and The Bladder Witch. I truly cherish those names and am always open to other suggestions as I feel they are one of the highest forms of compliment that I can receive. These women were so grateful that some of them even cried tears of joy after getting their lives back. That is why I do what I do. I am a Physical Therapist who has been treating women with urinary incontinence and overactive bladder for over fourteen years.

Let's get back to the Super Nanny. The Super Nanny believes in time-outs for children (and parents) who misbehave. Wouldn't that be great if we could do the same for our misbehaving bladders?

Instead, women end up putting *themselves* in time-out because they believe they have no other option. I wish I had a nickel for every time a woman said to me, "I don't want to end up like my grandmother."

The Progression

One day a woman starts wearing the occasional panty liner when she leaves her house. This quickly leads to her wearing panty liners every day. Next, she needs to buy the larger pads because the panty liners are no longer containing the leaks. Does this sound at all familiar?

In time, she may end up buying the pull-up style incontinence diapers because now she is doing several loads of laundry every day just to have clean clothes to wear. That does not sound too appealing, does it? Well, brace yourself: it can only go downhill from there.

She wakes up in the middle of the night just to realize that she wet the bed. It is now time to start wearing the pull-up style incontinence diapers both day and night. You see, it isn't bad enough that she has to wash three outfits a day ... now she has to wash three outfits a day and the bedding as well. But what happens when she starts leaking through those too? And there it is. She starts putting herself into time-outs.

She declines friends' invitations because she fears having an accident in public. Of course, she only fears this because she has already experienced the shame and humiliation of it one too many times. Entertaining at home is easier anyway, right? Then, one of those unexpected accidents occurs during a social gathering in her own home! So she stops inviting guests over altogether. And, traveling for leisure? Not on her life!

Eventually, she only leaves the house if it is absolutely necessary ... you know, like for groceries and more pads. Or better yet, she has a few close friends or family members do her shopping for her. But, what if that is not an option? What if she has no one to run errands for her? That is pretty much the final straw. Now it is time for someone else to take care of her. Hopefully it is an option for her to move in with a family member. But how long do you think her family will be able to handle her daily incontinent episodes? As hard as they try, everyone has their limits. That is when the only option left for her is a nursing home.

Although your incontinence may not have progressed this far, it may sound as though I am exaggerating the effects of urinary incontinence in our society, but I certainly am not. I have heard first-hand story after story after story of this exact situation happening to patients' loved ones. That is one of the most common fears that I hear during our sessions ... "I do not want to end up like my grandmother." It breaks my heart. All of this, however, can be corrected and even prevented with physical therapy!

The Solution

Helping women overcome urinary incontinence is my passion. It is my goal as a physical therapist, and has been for the past fourteen years, to help as many women as possible overcome urinary incontinence. I know it is a bold statement and that it sounds more like a pipe dream from the best-intentioned physical therapist. The fact is, however, that I have already cured the symptoms of incontinence for well over a thousand women. But I can only help seven or eight women a day overcome this devastating disease as a practicing physical therapist. As fabulous as that is, it is not enough ... for me. I have helped only a sliver of the women this problem affects.

Incontinence affects over 19 million women in the world today and it is one of the leading causes of nursing home admissions.

I believe what I am doing is a wonderful thing, but surely there is so much more that I can do. As a Taurus, I am extremely stubborn when it comes to getting what I want. As a perfectionist, I will never stop trying to come up with the perfect solution. In this case, what I want is to find the perfect solution to help hundreds of thousands, or even millions, of women all over the world get their lives back by taking control of their bladders. There are not enough hours in a day to individually cure that many women. Hence, this book is my solution. It holds the key to breaking the devastating cycle of urinary incontinence. Unlike other solutions, which just make your symptoms more tolerable, my techniques will **cure** your symptoms.

During my fourteen years of research, I came across a common theme: practically every book written about urinary incontinence and overactive bladder, although few, was written by a physician. Why is that? Unsure of the answer myself, I purchased a dozen of the most current books I could find (ranging in copyright year from 1989 to 2010) to see what they had to say. As far as I could tell, most of the physician-written books that I acquired on urinary incontinence followed the same general outline: definition of urinary incontinence, types of urinary incontinence, anatomy and physiology of the urinary tract system, urodynamic testing and invasive cystoscopic procedures, medications including possible side effects, and surgical interventions including possible complications. Interestingly enough, only one of the books mentioned physical therapy as an option. Unfortunately, it was just a couple of sentences out of the entire book, which made it easy to overlook.

The information in the books was educational, but nothing specifically addressed a cure. One book actually had a chapter on how to cope with symptoms of urinary incontinence. Physicians are the experts when it comes to knowing how the human body functions. But physical therapists are the experts when it comes to knowing how muscles function. That said, **the bladder is a muscle**. It is time to learn a fresh new approach to preventing and curing urinary incontinence, and we will do it without medications and without surgeries and we will do it together. So let us begin.

Chapter 2
Test-Taking 101

Before we get started, it would be helpful for you to fill out the following two forms. The information you record will be addressed later in the book. Keep in mind that we will readdress this and see all your progress.

The first form, the **Urinary Incontinence Impact Questionnaire**, will take no more than a few minutes to complete. This will be the starting point, or baseline, of your current symptoms. If one of your answers falls between two different numbers, then circle the larger number. Tally your points and then move on. Points will be addressed later in the book.

Urinary Incontinence Impact Questionnaire

Frequency of urinary leaks (small & large):	The longest time I can wait to pee is:
0 I do not leak at all	0 4 hours
1 I leak 1-3 times a month	1 3 1/2 hours
2 I leak 1-3 days a week	2 3 hours
3 I leak 4-6 days a week	3 2 1/2 hours
4 I leak 1-3 times a day	4 2 hours
5 I leak 3-6 times a day	5 1 1/2 hours
6 I leak more than 6 times a day	6 1 hour
7 I dribble all day long	7 1/2 hour or less
At most, I wear ____ pads in 24 hours:	The shortest time I can wait to pee is:
0 0	0 4 hours
1 1	1 3 1/2 hours
2 2	2 3 hours
3 3	3 2 1/2 hours
4 4	4 2 hours
5 5	5 1 1/2 hours
6 6	6 1 hour
7 More than 6	7 1/2 hour or less
I drink ____ glasses of fluid each day:	At most, I wake up ____ times at night to pee:
0 8 or more	0 0
1 7	1 1
2 6	2 2
3 5	3 3
4 4	4 4
5 3	5 5
6 2	6 6
7 Less than 2	7 More than 6
The types of protection I use are:	I leak with ____. (Circle all that apply)
0 None	0 N/A
1 Folded tissue paper	1 Cough, sneeze, laugh
2 Panty liners	1 Sports, exercise, running, jumping
3 Small pads	1 Getting out of bed
4 Medium pads	1 Getting out of a car
5 Large pads	1 Getting up from a chair
6 Two pads at the same time	1 The sound of running water
7 Pull-up style	1 Urgency or trying to get to the bathroom

Date: _____   Score: _____/56

Chapter 2: Test-Taking 101

The following is a sample of a completed Urinary Incontinence Impact Questionnaire.

Urinary Incontinence Impact Questionnaire

Frequency of urinary leaks (small & large):	The longest time I can wait to pee is:
0 I do not leak at all	0 4 hours
1 I leak 1-3 times a month	1 3 1/2 hours
2 I leak 1-3 days a week	2 3 hours
3 I leak 4-6 days a week	3 2 1/2 hours
4 I leak 1-3 times a day	**(4)** 2 hours
5 I leak 3-6 times a day	5 1 1/2 hours
(6) I leak more than 6 times a day	6 1 hour
7 I dribble all day long	7 1/2 hour or less

At most, I wear ____ pads in 24 hours:	The shortest time I can wait to pee is:
0 0	0 4 hours
1 1	1 3 1/2 hours
2 2	2 3 hours
3 3	3 2 1/2 hours
4 4	4 2 hours
(5) 5	5 1 1/2 hours
6 6	**(6)** 1 hour
7 More than 6	7 1/2 hour or less

I drink ____ glasses of fluid each day:	At most, I wake up ____ times at night to pee:
0 8 or more	0 0
1 7	1 1
2 6	2 2
3 5	3 3
(4) 4	**(4)** 4
5 3	5 5
6 2	6 6
7 Less than 2	7 More than 6

The types of protection I use are:	I leak with ____. (Circle all that apply)
0 None	0 N/A
1 Folded tissue paper	**(1)** Cough, sneeze, laugh
(2) Panty liners	1 Sports, exercise, running, jumping
3 Small pads	1 Getting out of bed
4 Medium pads	1 Getting out of a car
5 Large pads	**(1)** Getting up from a chair
6 Two pads at the same time	**(1)** The sound of running water
7 Pull-up style	**(1)** Urgency or trying to get to the bathroom

Date: 5/18/10   Score: 35 /56

The second form, the **Input & Output Diary**, will take you three days to complete. It is a three-day baseline recording of every time you drink something, every time you pee, and every time you have an accident, or leakage of urine. It should be recorded in chronological order and cover a 24-hour period for each of the three days. I have added an example of one of these diaries to help clarify your recording of information.

Input & Output Diary

Date	Time	Fluid Intake	Void in Toilet	Accident	Comments

Chapter 2: Test-Taking 101

The following is a sample of a completed Input & Output Diary. This condensed version will hopefully answer any unaddressed questions you may have about recording your information.

Input & Output Diary

Date	Time	Fluid Intake	Void in Toilet	Accident	Comments
5/18/10	11:45 pm		M		up at night to pee
5/19/10	1:45 am		M		up at night to pee
	2:20 am		S		up at night to pee
	5:00 am		M		up at night to pee
	7:00 am		S	S	on way to bathroom
	8:10 am	6 oz coffee			with caffeine
	8:15 am		S	M	sneezed
	9:00 am		S	S	on way to bathroom
	10:30 am	6 oz coffee		S	caffeine, stood up from chair
	11:45 am		M		
	1:15 pm		S		
	2:00 pm		S	S	on way to bathroom
	2:15 pm	8 oz milk			
	4:00 pm		M		
	4:30 pm	8 oz water			
	6:00 pm		M		
	7:00 pm		S	S	on way to bathroom
	8:10 pm		S		
	8:45 pm			S	stood up from chair
	9:00 pm		S		
	10:30 pm		S		bedtime

This diary does not need to be daunting. I will break it down into simple steps to make your job easier. Like everything in life, if you understand the pattern of the problem you can begin to find the solution in a simplified manner. For each entry, you will need to record the time.

Fluid Intake

Input & Output Diary

Date	Time	Fluid Intake	Void in Toilet	Accident	Comments
	8:10 am	6 oz coffee			with caffeine
	10:30 am	6 oz coffee			with caffeine
	2:15 pm	8 oz milk			

Please note the **Fluid Intake** column. This column is used to record both the amount and type of fluid you are drinking. Make sure you also record the time it occurred in the **Time** column.

When recording the amount of fluid, do your best to record the number of ounces for each drink. If it is in a kitchen glass or mug, measure how much it holds for an accurate recording. If you are unsure of the number of ounces, then use the classification of small, medium, or large when recording your drink. If it takes you a longer period to finish a drink, like a 16-ounce bottle of water, then record the start and stop times for that drink.

When recording the type of fluid you are drinking, be specific. If it is coffee, tea, or soda, make sure you record caffeine versus decaf. If it is juice, record the specific type. If the water has bubbles, record that too.

Void in Toilet

Input & Output Diary

Date	Time	Fluid Intake	Void in Toilet	Accident	Comments
	7:00 am		S		
	8:15 am		S		
	11:45 am		M		

Next, let's look at the **Void in Toilet** column. This column is used to record the amount of urine you pee both day and night. Make sure you also record the time it occurred in the **Time** column.

Use the classification of small, medium, or large for each time you urinate. A small amount might be when you have a strong urge to pee, but not much comes out, whereas a large amount might be your first pee of the morning.

Accident

Input & Output Diary

Date	Time	Fluid Intake	Void in Toilet	Accident	Comments
	8:15 am			M	sneezed
	9:00 am			M	on way to bathroom
	10:30 am			S	stood up from chair

Now, look at the **Accident** column. This column is used to record the amount of each unintentional loss of urine, otherwise known as a leak. Make sure you also record the time it occurred in the **Time** column as well as what you were doing in the **Comments** column.

You can use the classification of small, medium, or large to record the size of the leak. If it is just a few drops, then record it as small. If it filled the pad or made you change your clothes, then it may be a medium or a large.

Some women leak without realizing when it happened. If this is the case, then record the time you noticed it and then add a note in the **Comments** column as such.

Lastly, direct your attention to the **Comments** column. This column is used to record pieces of interesting information.

The following lists examples of information to be recorded here:

1. Record what time you got up for the day.
2. Record what time you went to bed.
3. Record how many times you got up at night to pee.
4. Record what you were doing if you leaked (coughing, standing up from a chair, rushing to the bathroom, etc.)
5. Record if you had any really strong urges to pee.
6. Record if you peed 'just in case' to avoid a potential leak (before leaving the house, before exercise, before a long car ride, etc.)

These will be useful pieces of information later in the book when I teach you how to analyze your diary.

Your completed version will probably be two to four pages in length. Although it is a bit of a pain to fill out, it is a highly effective training tool I use to explain individual leaking occurrences. Once you complete your diary, put it aside for later use.

You are now ready to begin the journey. All you have to do is turn the page. Enjoy the trip!

Chapter 3
Muscle Power

Let's talk about what's going on with the bladder, why it is acting as it is, and how it should act. In order to fix it, we need to know what is wrong with it and how it should be working.

The bladder is a muscle. But, unlike most muscles, the bladder should be 'at rest' 99% of the time in each 24-hour period. 'At rest' means the bladder is filling and stretching to accommodate urine and fluids, but it is **not** contracting. The remaining 1% of the time is when the bladder should contract. Contractions should **only** occur when you are sitting on the toilet to pee **and** at a *convenient* time for you. Only then should the bladder contract to push the urine out of your body and into the toilet. Once empty, it is time for the bladder to rest (stretch and fill) again.

The kidneys make the urine, and the urine gets stored in the bladder. This makes the bladder the urine's 'holding tank.' As the bladder fills with urine, it slowly expands in size like a balloon filling with water (i.e., a resting bladder). While resting, the bladder is able to stretch until it becomes full of fluid. This filling and stretching process should take about four hours. When it is almost full, the bladder sends a message to the brain that says, "I'm pretty full, so you better let her know." That is when you get the signal from your brain that it is time to head for the bathroom to empty your bladder.

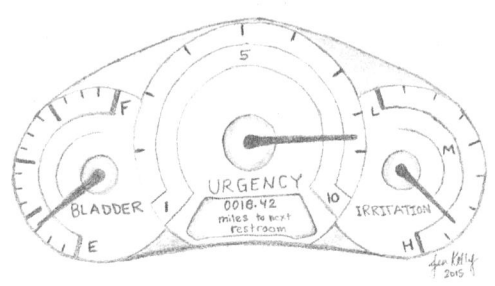

Although you received a signal, it is important to realize that your bladder is still at rest. Think of the bladder like the gasoline tank in your car. A car's dashboard light signals when the gas tank is almost empty. 'Almost empty' means you have enough time to get to a gas station before you run out of gas. Your bladder signals you similarly, but also allows you enough time to make it to the bathroom before it starts contracting and emptying.

This signal that you receive from your brain should be a normal, casual signal, which means the bladder has not contracted yet and is still at rest. It should **not** be an "Oh my God, I have to pee now!" signal. Many times, this casual signal is quite easy to ignore. Maybe you are in the middle of an important phone call and stopping now would be very inconvenient for you. Therefore, you continue chatting. After all, you still have time to get to the bathroom.

Before you realize it, another half hour has passed. Then comes the gentle reminder signal again from your bladder and brain telling you that you have to pee. Since now is a good time, you decide to go to the bathroom. At this point, the bladder is still at rest.

You walk to the bathroom, and your bladder is still at rest. You unbutton your pants, and your bladder is still at rest. You sit down on the toilet, and your bladder is still at rest. As you begin to pee, that is when the brain sends a message to your bladder saying, "OK, she's ready. Go ahead and contract." Now the bladder is contracting to rid itself of the urine.

CHAPTER 3: MUSCLE POWER

The bladder should only contract when you are intentionally peeing. After it empties out all of the urine, it returns to its resting state, and the four-hour filling process begins again. It is important to remember that the only time the bladder should contract is when *you* initiate the void, and no sooner. If the bladder contracts at any other time of the day or night, then you get the following symptoms; urinary frequency (peeing too often), urinary urgency (needing to get to the bathroom NOW or you might leak), and urinary incontinence (the leaking of urine, one drop or a lot).

Since the bladder should take about four hours to fill, this means that a normal bladder should only empty five to seven times in a 24-hour period. At most, only one of those five to seven times should be at night, but that certainly is not the norm.

I would like you to meet Judy. Judy is a 44-year-old mother of three teenage children. She has a very busy day planned, but today she is extremely tired. Last night was a bad night. For no apparent reason, Judy woke up four times to pee instead of her usual three. What a horrible night!

Once she finally got the kids off to school, Judy jumped into the shower. The warm steamy water always makes her feel better. Just as she is about to pick up the soap, she starts to leak urine. "What the hell was that?" she wonders. Well, at least she was in the shower, so cleanup was a breeze.

After she gets dressed, she heads to the kitchen and pours a hot cup of coffee, sits in her favorite chair and begins planning her busy day. Her list complete, she stands up to grab another cup of coffee. Today is definitely a two-cup-of-coffee-kind-of-day, maybe even three! On the way to the kitchen, Judy suddenly is gripped by a very strong urge to pee. "Oh, for crying out loud ... not again!" is what she says as she hurries towards the bathroom.

As she races towards the bathroom, the urge grows stronger. She starts thinking, "Oh my God, I'm not

17

going to make it." Seconds later, she is finally in the bathroom. She begins squirming as she fumbles with the buttons on her pants. "Note to self ... buy elastic waist pants!" After no small feat, they are undone and yes, she is going to make it this time. She starts pulling down her pants and, yes, yes ... NO! Dammit! Out comes the pee! She was so close to making it this time ... again. Guess she can add those undies to the laundry ... again. Time to put on a panty liner ... AGAIN!

For all you women who have not begun leaking but have already found yourselves wondering where the next bathroom is located, prevention is of the utmost importance. Be assured, if you do not intervene immediately, it will be you trying to make it to the bathroom without leaking.

Should you be one of the unfortunate ones who is already experiencing episodes of leaking, it does not have to become a bigger problem. Whether your leaks are small or large, there is so much you can do to help stop the progression and even cure your symptoms of this horribly debilitating problem.

The beginning of the progression for most women is the phase where it is 'not so bad.' They never associate themselves at this point with leaking and **never** with incontinence. But know this–**one drop is a leak!**

Chapter 4
One Drop Is A Leak

It is normal for the bladder to contract.
It is not normal for the bladder to shrink.

A normal bladder should empty every four or more hours, or five to seven times each day. If, for any reason, a bladder starts emptying more than eight times a day on a regular basis, it starts to shrink (as in Judy's case). The bladder shrinks because **the bladder is a muscle.**

Have you ever known someone who broke an arm? My oldest son, Max, did when he was eight years old. He fell from the monkey bars at the park and landed directly on his elbow. He wore a cast for four weeks, one that kept his elbow at a 90-degree angle. During those four weeks, Max was unable to straighten his arm. When the cast was finally removed, he was able to straighten his arm but not all the way. Why was that? Because the muscles that allow his arm to straighten fully had shrunk.

You see, muscles are very smart and love to be efficient. They will also do whatever is necessary in order to stay that way. Since Max was unable to straighten his arm, his muscles were unable to access their full length. Muscles know that when they cannot access their full length then they are no longer as strong or as efficient as they once were. Muscles find this, of course, unacceptable. Max's muscles, to remedy this, decided to become physically shorter by actively ridding themselves of some of their unused muscle fibers. In turn, this would allow them to have a new length (a shorter one) so they would again become strong and efficient despite their loss. Muscles truly are amazing!

The bladder is a muscle. The bladder is most efficient when it is allowed to stretch to its maximum capacity, which is at about 4 hours of filling. What if the bladder is emptied after only two hours of filling? Maybe you were going to the grocery store and thought, "I'd better pee now, so I don't have to pee half way through grocery shopping." Or, what if you get that sudden urge to pee, even though you just peed an hour ago? These occurrences add up and before you know it, the bladder is no longer allowed to stretch for the full four hours that it should. The bladder then becomes inefficient.

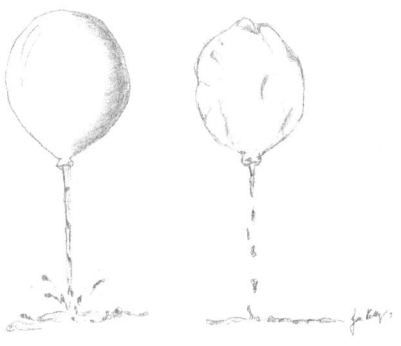

Picture a balloon **full** of water, and imagine I am holding the end of it closed. If I open the end of the balloon, then the water will come out at a good rate. But what if I take that same balloon and only half fill it with water? Then when I open the end of it the water will only trickle out (i.e., come out at a slower rate). The same principle applies to the bladder. If the bladder contracts when it is full, then the fluid will come out at a good rate. If the bladder contracts when it is only half full, then it will come out at a slower rate. The bladder considers this slower rate of elimination as inefficient.

To remedy this, it decides to lose muscle fibers so that it can become smaller. What was once a half-full bladder at the larger size is now a full bladder at a smaller size. Again, this makes the rate of elimination quicker, which makes the bladder more efficient. It's a win-win situation for the bladder, but a lose-lose situation for you. Emptying your bladder before going to the grocery store seemed quite convenient at the time. Having to empty your bladder in the middle of a fantastic movie at the theater? Not so convenient!

It does not end there though. You see, since you are now peeing more than eight times in a 24 hour period on a regular basis, you will find yourself waking up to pee in the middle of the night as well.

Everything slows down when you sleep; your respiratory rate, your heart rate, your production of urine. Since the kidneys produce urine at a slower rate when you are sleeping, then the bladder fills at a slower rate. In general, the bladder takes twice as long to fill at night as it does during the day. Therefore, if you can wait four hours between peeing in the daytime <u>on a regular basis,</u> then you should get an eight-hour straight night before your bladder wakes you up to empty. Unfortunately, this also means that if you pee every hour (consistently) during the day, you most likely will be up every two hours to pee at night. Also, if your time between voids varies throughout each day, then so will your number of jaunts to the bathroom at night.

It starts with one time but quickly works its way to four, five, or even six times out of bed each night to pee. Your bladder is happy since it is again efficient, but you, on the other hand, could use a good night's sleep.

Our bladders may be the culprits, but make no mistake: we are their accomplices. It's a wicked web, my friend!

Chapter 5
You Irritate Me

The bladder can get irritated. This happened to Judy, who eventually spent a good part of her day running to the bathroom or leaking urine. Sometimes I can get irritated. When I do, I feel like I want to jump out of my skin and scream. I like to think of the bladder this way as well, only to a lesser degree.

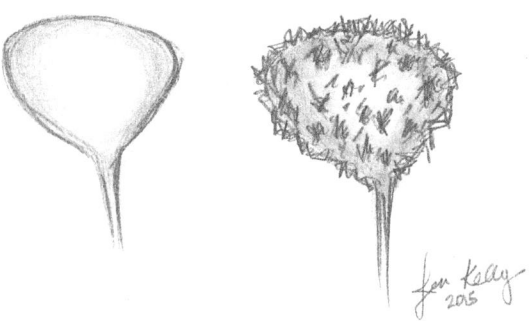

When the bladder is irritated, think of its inner walls as being itchy and twitchy. These itchy, twitchy inner walls cause the entire bladder, inside and out, to contract. Remember, the bladder should only contract when you are intentionally voiding. If it contracts at any other time, those contractions are considered unwanted because they cause you to pee too frequently, to run urgently to the bathroom, and to leak urine. As a result, a calm bladder should ultimately be our goal.

There are dozens of ways a bladder can get irritated. It would be nearly impossible to avoid all of the things that irritate the bladder and, to be honest, quite ridiculous of me to ask anyone to try even. I prefer to keep the *Don't Do* list short and simple by having you avoid only, within reason, the most irritating of all bladder irritants, at least initially. This smaller list will not only improve your ability to follow my program, but will also improve your success rate in ending your bladder problems in the least amount of time possible.

In essence, it's downright easy to follow and extremely effective in a very short amount of time. It sounds too good to be true, doesn't it? Well, it's not! The fact is, in a matter of days, your symptoms **will** begin to dissipate just by following my very simple program.

For years, your bladder has been able to process and neutralize all of the fluids you gave it whether they were 'good fluids' or 'irritating fluids,' and you were none the wiser. Unfortunately for you, your bladder is now tired, frustrated, and feeling very much overworked. You see, no matter how hard it works to neutralize the irritants, which takes extra energy, the irritants just keep coming. So one day your bladder throws its proverbial arms up in the air and says, "I'm done! This is your problem now!" And there you are, all of a sudden, running to the bathroom because you have to pee. Apparently what comes around **does** go around! Our job now becomes keeping our bladders calm. But how do we do this?

Ultimately, a doctor's job is to teach us how to stay healthy. One of the standard recommendations is that we should drink at least eight 8-ounce glasses of water each day. We know water is good for us, and we certainly trust our doctors, but how many of us really drink that much water? Certainly not many of the people I know. Why is that? Could it be the negative consequences associated with limited water intake, whatever they may be, are not great enough for us to worry? God knows we certainly have enough to worry about on a daily basis already.

What if, however, the doctor told us if we don't drink eight 8-ounce glasses of water every day, then our hearts will stop beating, and we will die? I bet that would get our attention. I know it would certainly get mine! Fortunately for us, that is not the case. So, how bad could it actually be if we don't drink all that water? Obviously, not bad enough or the doctors would have told us, right?

The most common reason I hear from women for limiting their fluid intake (particularly water) is that they are convinced of the following; the more fluid they drink, the more they will pee and leak. So, what consequence do you think is worse for these women; the eventual unknown consequence of not drinking enough water **or** the fear their current bladder symptoms will worsen? Clearly that's a no-brainer!

Consequential fear is a powerful decision maker. Unfortunately, many of our choices are based on irrationally perceived consequences. I believe to make a sound decision we need to be rational, and we cannot be rational if we know not of which we speak.

The educational component of my program is paramount in curing bladder problems, just as it is during my physical therapy sessions. The truth is this: knowledge can set you free. Every woman I treat for bladder problems has the same irrational consequential fear that the more they drink, the more they will pee or leak. Let me dispel your fears about the effects of fluid intake on the bladder. Once done, you will have the information you need in order to make a sound decision regarding the amount of fluid you should, or should not, drink each day.

Fact ... our bodies need to consume eight 'good fluids' each day, evenly spaced at least eight different times, to mix with our urine so our urine is not too strong. This diluted urine does not irritate the bladder, but rather keeps its environment neutral and calm. A calm bladder is a content bladder. As a result, a content bladder is able to hold in its urine for a longer period of time.

Concentrated urine (strong and yellow) irritates the bladder. An irritated bladder is annoyed (itchy and twitchy) so it contracts sooner than it should to rid itself of the irritant.

CHAPTER 5: YOU IRRITATE ME

GOOD FLUIDS VS. IRRITATING FLUIDS

Good fluids are any type of fluid that does not irritate the bladder. Water is, of course, one of the good fluids. Irritating fluids are any type of fluid that irritates the bladder, otherwise known as bladder irritants. Knowing the difference between these two types of fluids will make all the difference in your progress. Listed below are the different types of good fluids (a.k.a., 'Lucky Liquids') you may choose. Keep in mind that any drink used to replace a meal (protein drinks, smoothies, etc.) does not count as one of your eight daily fluids.

<u>The Lucky Liquids</u>

1. Water, hot or cold
2. Milk or milk alternative (almond, coconut, soy, etc.)
3. Decaffeinated coffee, hot or iced
4. Decaffeinated tea, hot or iced
5. Flavored water, no bubbles
6. Real fruit added to water for flavoring
7. Non-acidic juices like apple, grape, berry and other fruit flavors

Bladder irritants are hidden in the foods or drinks you have every day. They don't necessarily have to be bad for you, but they certainly can throw the bladder into a tailspin of embarrassing symptoms. I have comprised a list of irritants I like to refer to as 'The Ferocious Four.' Memorize these, and it will serve you well for years to come.

<u>The Ferocious Four</u>

1. Caffeine (Coffee, Tea, Soda, Energy Drinks)
2. Alcohol (Wine, Beer, Liquor)
3. Carbonation (Soda, Tonic, Bubbly Water)
4. Acidic Drinks (OJ, Grapefruit Juice, Tomato/V8 Juice, Lemonade)

By drinking these fluids on a regular basis, you are essentially making your bladder contract when it should be at rest. Trying to calm it back down will now be all up to you.

There are foods that irritate the bladder, but over the years I have found their impact on the bladder to be of little concern. Spicy foods, tomatoes, and foods with aspartame if eaten daily, however, can certainly irritate the bladder as well.

Maybe you are one of the few who rarely drinks any of the Ferocious Four. Then why are you still suffering from these symptoms? Could there be another explanation? Here comes the answer that everyone hates to hear; 'it depends'. Just let me explain. Although there certainly are other reasons for leaking, the most likely reason is the fifth type of bladder irritant or, as I like to call it, the **Invisible Irritant**.

Water (or any other 'good fluid') is the Invisible Irritant, but it is only an irritant when it is **not** there. Without water or other good fluids, the urine in the bladder is too strong and concentrated and thus irritates the bladder. It presents as a strong smelling, yellow urine when you pee. Therefore, clearer pee means a calmer bladder.

THE LESS YOU DRINK, THE MORE YOU PEE.

For some reason, water is the liquid that most women tend to avoid because 'if they drink it, they will just have to pee.' I cannot begin to tell you how many times I have heard that or some variation of it. So, for all of you out there who are intentionally limiting your fluid intake on a daily basis so that you wont have to pee as often, **STOP!** What you are actually doing is the opposite: you are irritating your bladder and making yourself pee more often **because** you are not drinking enough good fluids.

Limiting your fluid intake creates a concentrated environment in your bladder. It contracts when it should not. It causes you to feel the urge to pee when you should not.

The more you drink, the less you pee.

You must drink at least 65-70 fluid ounces of good fluids each day to allow your bladder to wait the necessary four hours between pees. This amount is manageable. It is roughly eight 8-ounce drinks a day, just like the doctor ordered. That's only one drink every one and a half to two hours, and it does not have to be just water. Any combination of the good fluids totaling 65-70 fluid ounces each day is acceptable.

Eight ounces is much less fluid than you think. A one-cup measuring cup holds eight ounces. A child's juice box holds eight ounces. A Dixie cup holds eight ounces. An average bottle of water, 16.9 ounces, holds two of your eight-ounce daily drinks!

These good fluids help to dilute the urine. The more diluted the urine, the longer it will stay in the bladder because the bladder will not be irritated. The longer it stays in the bladder, the less you will have to pee.

Your bladder is happy when it is full of good fluids. It does not feel itchy and twitchy. It does not feel the need to contract. It does not make you pee! If you don't do what the doctor says, then at least do what the physical therapist says; drink your fluids for your bladder's sake and, in return, your bladder will set you free!

Chapter 6
The Truth About Poop

Some bladder leaks are caused by the bowels.

Constipation is a big deal! In fact, it can affect urinary frequency, urinary urgency, urinary leakage, and organ prolapse. Since a picture is worth a thousand words, that is where we shall begin.

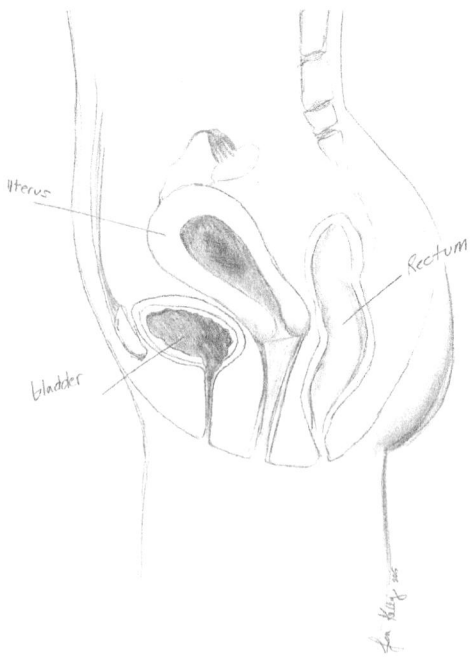

CHAPTER 6: THE TRUTH ABOUT POOP

Notice in the cross section above the proximity of the bowels to the bladder. Now, look down at your stomach and pelvis. How the heck can all of that be happening in such a small amount of space?

The Bowels

The bowels consist of the small and large intestines, which are continuous connections of tubes running from the stomach to the anus. Although pretty straightforward, the surprise lies in the overall length.

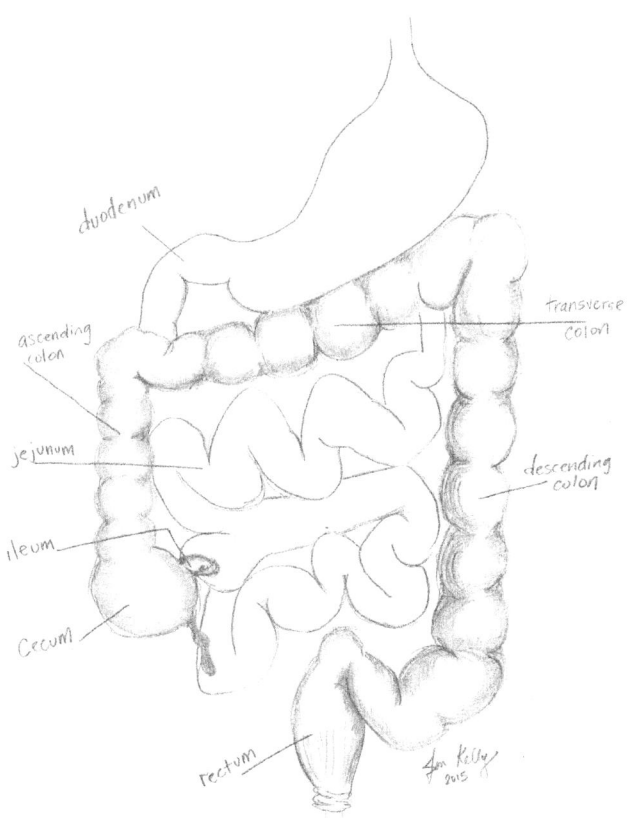

THE ART OF CONTROL

A. The three components of the small intestine add up to 22 feet in length

1. Duodenum
2. Jejunum
3. Ileum

B. The three components of the large intestine add up to five feet in length

1. Cecum
2. Colon
3. Rectum

When you add the small and large intestine, the total length is 27 feet. That is four to five times the length of your entire body! And, it is all shoved in that tiny space between your stomach and your anus. Holy crap! (No pun intended.)

Now, let's assume your bowels are full. The picture might resemble something like this:

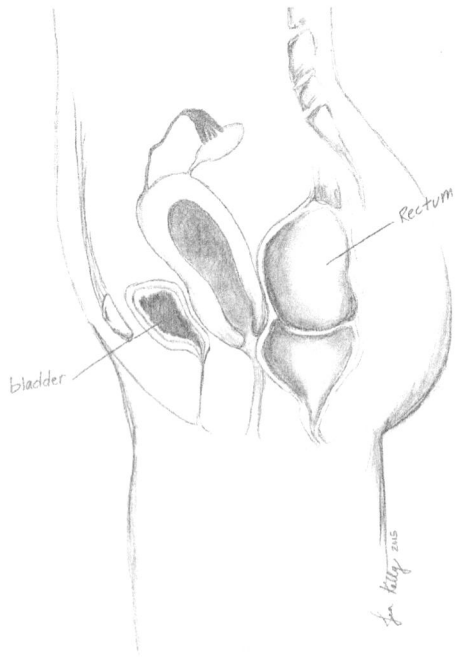

30

Notice how the full bowels push against the bladder. This added pressure can limit the bladder's ability to fill effectively to capacity that, in turn, can affect its ability to fully empty. This leads to leaks and even potential infection.

Picture again the bladder like a balloon filling with water.

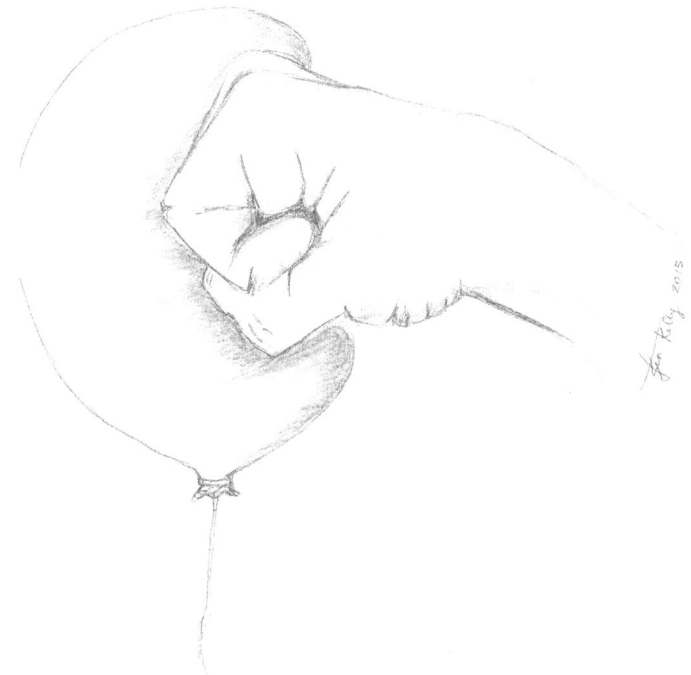

Now let's take a closer look to see how this added pressure causes the bladder to misbehave.

Urinary Frequency

When the bladder is unable to expand to its fullest potential, it can be forced to empty sooner and more *frequently* than it should. Although it might be a normal, calm signal, it still should not be happening so soon.

Urinary Urgency

Irritating fluids can cause bladder contractions and urinary urgency. Remember, if the fluids are too irritating to the bladder (the Ferocious Four or the Invisible Irritant), they can cause unwanted, *urgent* bladder contractions.

For example, let's say your bladder can hold a maximum of 32 fluid ounces. If eight of those 32 ounces were from caffeinated coffee, then one-fourth of your bladder would contain irritating fluids. However, the bladder can handle a small amount of irritating fluid without necessarily causing you problems.

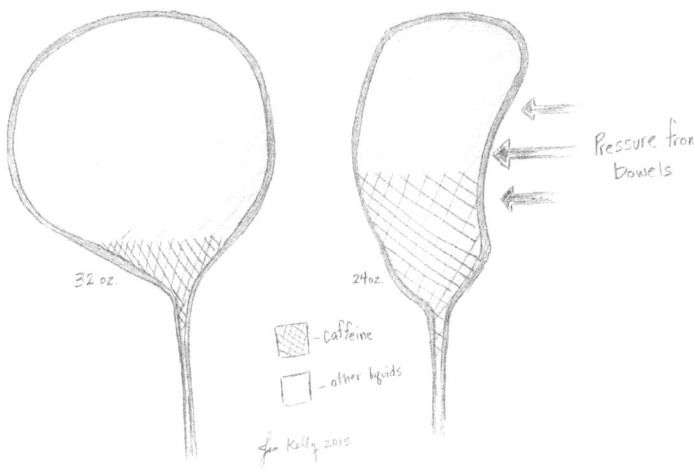

But, if you happen to be temporarily constipated, your bowels will push on your bladder. Now your bladder might only hold a total of 24 fluid ounces instead of its usual 32 ounces because of constipation.

Unfortunately for you, that same eight-ounce cup of caffeinated coffee now irritates one-third of your entire bladder instead of only one-fourth of it.

Now the caffeine has a larger impact on your bladder. At that higher level of irritation, the bladder is more likely to respond with an *urgent* signal to empty.

Even though the size of that coffee, or the amount of caffeine in it, has not changed at all, it is actually now more irritating to the bladder when you are constipated.

Add to that the potential of a long history of constipation (which is extremely common) and over time the bladder shrinks, just as we will learn in Chapter 7, The Constipation Revelation.

The combination of a smaller bladder and full bowels is a recipe for bladder disaster. What used to be a normal, calm signal to void is now a sudden, strong, *urgent* signal. And, hopefully, you will still make it to the bathroom in time!

Urinary Leakage

In addition to the above urinary problems, added pressure from full bowels can also cause urinary leakage. Some leaks from constipation are due to an irritated bladder while other leaks are caused by direct pressure on the bladder.

Irritated Bladder

Just as an irritated bladder can lead to urinary leakage, your chances of leaking increase when you are constipated because of the added pressure on the bladder.

Direct Pressure

Leakage from direct pressure on a bladder is a little more subtle. When you cough, sneeze, or laugh, there is an immediate force of pressure placed on the bladder that comes from the abdominal cavity above. It is hard enough to overcome that amount of pressure without leaking, but add to that the full bowels pushing against the bladder and your risk of leaking increases even more.

Standing up from a chair or getting out of a bed are a few more examples of direct pressure on a bladder. Good body mechanics, however, can prevent this (see Chapter 16, FAQs & Tricks Of The Trade).

If you do not use the proper body mechanics while standing up or getting out of bed, you actually end up squashing the bladder because you are bending over too far.

Know this: all of the above potential leaks could probably have been prevented if the bowels had not been full or backed up. That is not to say that every leak is caused by full bowels, but certainly many of them are.

Organ Prolapse–I've fallen, and I can't get up

A prolapsed organ has fallen or slipped out of place. In addition to problems with frequency, urgency, and leakage, that long history of constipation can also be a cause of organ prolapse (bladder, uterus, rectum, vagina or a combination of prolapses). Once that occurs, your risk increases for urinary frequency, urinary urgency, bladder leakage and discomfort.

There are different levels of severity for prolapses, the most severe corrected only by surgery. You can prevent this with both pelvic floor exercise (see Chapter 12, The Inside Workout) and body mechanics training (see chapter 16, FAQs & Tricks Of The Trade).

In order to keep the bladder safe from all the potential effects of backed-up bowels, it is essential to keep the bowels moving. There are a few easy tricks I will share with you in the following chapter to do just that. Trust me, both your bowels and bladder will love you for it!

Chapter 7
The Constipation Revelation

Up to 28% of all women suffer from constipation. Although constipation is as prevalent as urinary incontinence in women, it seems to be much less talked about. It is for this reason most women I treat do not even realize they are constipated. Judy was one of those women.

Her bladder symptoms were exacerbated by her constipation, which, if unaddressed, would have resulted in less than perfect outcomes. One of the most difficult concepts for many to grasp is that constipation can occur despite having a bowel movement every day.

Constipation is having two or more of the following symptoms for a period of at least three months:

1. Having fewer than three bowel movements in one week
2. Having to strain when trying to evacuate stools
3. Having hard or lumpy stools
4. Having incomplete evacuation of stools
5. Having to manually evacuate your stools

I don't know about you, but that pretty much has been my life for the past thirty plus years. Well, it *had* been until I figured out how to address it.

There are many causes of constipation: medication side effects, poor bowel habits, low fiber diets, laxative overuse, hormonal disorders, limited daily fluid intake, colonic inertia, and pelvic floor dysfunction. Despite the long list, there *are* some simple techniques you can use to help counter its effects.

First, make sure you drink **all** your recommended daily fluid because your bowels need fluid too! The 65-70 fluid ounces of water (or good fluids) needed for your bladder is also necessary for your bowels to function properly. Without the moisture, it is like trying to pass a baseball through a keyhole! That doesn't sound like a whole lot of fun, does it? And remember: make sure you spread your fluids out evenly throughout the day.

The most common foods that cause constipation are:

1. Dairy (cheese, ice-cream)
2. Red meat
3. Processed foods (any packaged foods)
4. Foods containing wheat (pastas, cookies, cakes, donuts, and things with crusts like pizza–instead, try gluten free foods)
5. Foods high in fat (chips and fried foods)
6. Caffeine (it is dehydrating)

Limiting these foods is wise. You can still have these foods occasionally, but they certainly should not be part of your daily routine or a staple in your pantry.

Next, try adding more fiber to your diet like fruits and vegetables (preferably with the skins still on), grains, nuts, seeds, peas, and beans. They are chock-full of the kind of fiber your bowels crave and your bowels will surely thank you for it.

I understand how difficult it is to change dietary habits in today's uber-busy lifestyle. In addition to healthier foods being more expensive, everything is *'hurry up and get it done'*. The lunches need to be made, the kids need to get to school and to extracurricular activities, the boss needs you to complete the work of three people in 40 hours a week, the family wants to have a reunion at your house, the house needs a new roof, etc. There seems to be no time to relax anymore. Even planning a family vacation is craziness.

The fluid component of these recommendations, however, should already be a part of your life because you are hopefully already addressing that for your bladder. Do the best you can with what you have. Make small changes weekly and they will definitely add up over time to help regulate your bowels as well.

While working on the dietary changes, you can try a technique for a more immediate effect to relieve your bowels. I first learned about *positional voiding* while taking a course on pediatric bowel and bladder dysfunctions and treatments. It made so much sense I added it to my treatment regimen for adults.

The position in which you sit for a bowel movement can make a huge difference during bowel elimination. Try this:

1. Place a footstool at the base of your toilet. When you sit down, place your feet on the footstool so your knees are higher than your hips.
2. Spread your feet far apart so your legs, when looking at them, create the letter 'V'.
3. Rest your forearms on your thighs and relax. Yes, you should sit like a man!
4. Avoid straining (holding your breath while you push) to eliminate your bowels.
5. Time your bowel movement for 20 minutes after a meal since that is when the bowels are naturally stimulated to contract (peristalsis) and move things along.

These above five steps should be used every time you need to eliminate your bowels. Let me explain, in further detail, the reasons for their importance.

Footstool and Forearms (#1 and #2)

When your knees are higher than your hips, your pelvis is forced into a posterior pelvic tilt. During a posterior pelvic tilt, your anus is closer to the front of your body. Resting your forearms on your legs helps to reinforce this position by inducing relaxation of the muscles surrounding your pelvis. The path the bowel movement takes to leave your body is in a straighter line, making it easier to eliminate your bowels.

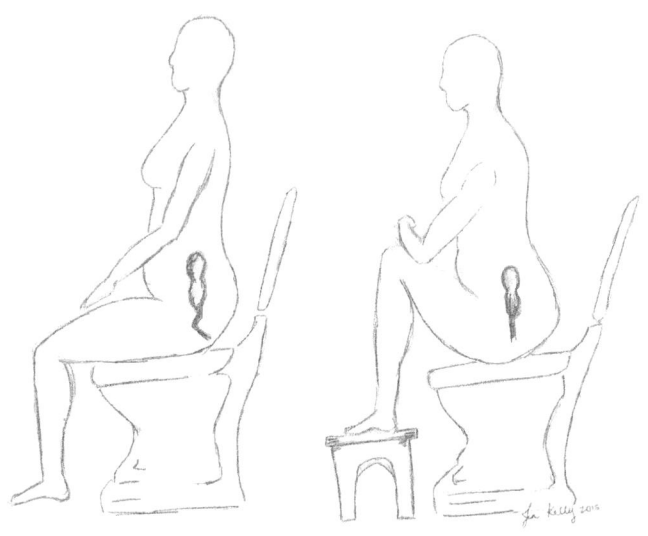

Conversely, when your knees are lower than your hips (when you have no footstool), then your anus is closer to the back of your body. Now the bowel movement has a little curve to round before leaving your body, making it more difficult to eliminate your bowels.

The Big 'V' (#3)

When your legs are far apart, in the position of the letter 'V,' you are 'opening up' or relaxing your pelvic floor muscles. When your legs are close together, you are 'closing' or tightening your pelvic floor muscles.

There is a close relationship between your pelvic floor muscles and your bowels and bladder. When the pelvic floor muscles are *contracting*, the bowels and bladder need to be at *rest*. This contraction helps prevent the unwanted loss of pee, poop, and gas.

Chapter 7: The Constipation Revelation

The same pelvic floor muscles that *contract* to prevent leaks *now need to be at rest* to allow your bowels and bladder to empty.

It really is a nice relationship, unless one of them decides to break the rules! Therefore, having your legs in a big 'V' is the key to having an easier, more successful, bowel movement.

Your pelvic floor muscles are postural muscles; their job is to: a) support your pelvic organs and b) keep pee, poop, and gas where it belongs. They are contracting all the time just like the muscles of your trunk and spine, which keep you upright. If your postural muscles stopped contracting right now, you would slump over like a wet noodle.

Avoid Straining (#4)

Constipation causes many of us to hold our breath when trying to have a bowel movement.

When we hold our breath and bear down to have a bowel movement, it forces pressure into our abdominal cavity. When we do not exhale, the pressure gets trapped in there. It pushes down with such force it can move our organs out of place (prolapse).

If this happens, our bladder and bowel symptoms can become much worse; larger bladder leaks, bowel leaks, and pain.

I have known many women who came to me with a diagnosis of prolapse. During the history of an evaluation of one woman, she told me she actually felt it happen. She was straining to eliminate her bowels, was unsuccessful, but felt something drop. She grabbed a mirror, looked at herself, and saw a bulge. Her prolapse was so severe that she could see one of her organs on the outside of her body. She was horrified. She pushed so hard she gave herself a prolapse. This organ could have been her bladder, her uterus, or even her rectum!

So *please, please* do not strain to have a bowel movement. Usually straining happens simultaneously when you hold your breath, and breath holding can result in a prolapse. If you must help to start your bowels moving, make sure you **exhale** as you push (and I use the term 'push' lightly).

If you must, you should exhale when you push. That will allow your abdominal muscles (belly muscles) to assist, which should be ok. As long as you are not forcing pressure down through your abdominal cavity with no place for it to exit, your organs should be safe. Remember, **exhale**!

Time Your BMs (#5)

With a little bit of coaxing, our bowels *will* behave. Poop travels through the bowels using peristalsis or bowel contractions. Although peristalsis is an involuntary action (meaning we cannot control it), there *is* something we can do to help it work in our favor to have a successful bowel movement.

Peristalsis naturally occurs 20 minutes after a meal. If we take that opportunity to sit down on the toilet (with the proper voiding posture as stated above), then those natural bowel contractions can help us empty our bowels.

Unfortunately, most of us are usually in such a hurry we miss that opportunity. Even worse, most of us do not even realize that opportunity exists.

I can even take that one step further and tell you our bowels can be trained to empty at the same time each day using this same technique. Just pick a meal, any meal, and begin the process! I am partial to bowel movements after dinner, as that is the time of day I am most able to relax. Give it a try for a few weeks and see what happens. You'll be amazed at what you will find.

When done, each of these techniques will help you stabilize your bowels. Once your bowels are stable, the potential leaks or prolapses associated with them will be non-existent!

Chapter 8
It's About Time

Three key components of my program are: **how much** you drink, **what** you drink, and **when** you drink it. These are all equally important in creating and maintaining a calm bladder environment. Chapter 5, You Irritate Me, detailed how much fluid you should drink.

How much you drink √

What You Drink

Now that you understand the amount of fluid required so your bladder can stay calm let's make sure it is the correct type of fluid. The fluids you drink must be **good fluids** or non-irritating fluids. As such, you cannot count caffeine, alcohol, and carbonated or acidic drinks (The Ferocious Four from Chapter 5, You Irritate Me). This list sounds like a lot to eliminate from your diet, but there are wonderful substitutes. Here is the list of good fluids called '**The Lucky Liquids**' introduced in Chapter 5, You Irritate Me, as well. Water lover or not, your options are numerous.

The Lucky Liquids

1. Water, hot or cold
2. Milk
3. Soy, coconut, almond or rice drinks
4. Decaffeinated coffee, hot or iced

5. Decaffeinated tea, hot or iced
6. Flavored water, no bubbles
7. Real fruit added to water for flavoring
8. Non-acidic juices like apple, grape, berry and other fruit flavors

It is important to understand that any combination of The Lucky Liquids may be used towards your daily fluid intake. Although water is the best choice for your bladder, and the least expensive, any of the above liquids will work. If you enjoy water then by all means drink water.

For those of you wondering if a cup of caffeinated coffee (or other favorite irritant) is still on the menu, rest assured. I discuss it specifically in Chapter 16, FAQs & Tricks of the Trade. As for now, try stocking up on a variety of The Lucky Liquids and see how quickly *your* luck will change!

How much you drink √
What you drink √

When You Drink

In order to establish a relaxed, calm, and neutral environment inside the bladder we need to create a habit to ensure the bladder fills at a constant rate. Sure this may take some time and energy but, again, not nearly as much as you may think.

The bladder works best when it has a *consistent* fluid flow entering it (rate of fill). Please realize you could take a whole course on how the bladder functions, and there is nothing simple about it. For simplicity's sake, however, let's assume it works as follows:

BLADDER'S RATE OF FILL = INPUT OF URINE + INPUT OF DRINKS

Since the kidneys produce urine at a constant rate, you need only concern yourself with the rate at which you drink your fluids. The slower or faster you drink your fluids, the slower or faster the bladder will fill. Therefore, we can alter the previous statement as follows:

Bladder's Rate of Fill = Input of Drinks

For example, let's say you are filling a balloon with water from your kitchen faucet. If you turn the faucet on low, the balloon will fill very slowly. If, however, you turn the faucet on high, the balloon will fill at a much faster rate. Essentially, this is what happens to the bladder as you drink fluids.

The goal is to have fluids enter the bladder **over** a consistent amount of time in order for fluids to exit the bladder **after** a consistent amount of time. For instance, if you want the bladder to empty every four hours (which you do), you will need to make sure that it fills at a **very consistent rate** over those same four hours. For this to happen you will need to drink about eight ounces of fluid every one and a half to two hours throughout the day. This will keep the urine *diluted* and ensure a relaxed, calm, and neutral environment inside the bladder.

I understand you will find this challenging for two reasons; 1) you do not get thirsty and 2) you are afraid if you drink more fluids you will pee and leak more. Trust me, this is not the case!

Your body, although it works best with the amount of fluid I have already recommended, has learned to live without it. Since your body no longer registers the feeling of thirst under normal circumstances, it cannot remind you when it is time to drink.

Therefore, it will be up to you initially to find a way to remember to drink your fluids throughout each day. Once you have established a good routine (see Chapter 16, FAQs & Tricks Of The Trade), you will be able to rely on your body once again. It will let you know when you are thirsty by *reminding* you when it needs fluids. Drinking fluids will no longer be an effort. It will be a habit.

How much you drink √
What you drink √
When you drink √

CHAPTER 9
RUSH HOUR

I would like you to meet Mary. Mary is a teacher at a middle school and has been for many years. She loves her job, especially the kids. They are a great bunch, always keeping her on her toes and always making her laugh.

For the past several years, Mary has been having a lot of difficulty with her bladder. For some reason, she is finding it harder and harder to wait until the end of her classes to go to the bathroom. She often gets a sudden urge to pee without any warning. When these urges occur, her instinct is to hurry to the bathroom before she has an accident. Thankfully this technique works for her because, so far, she has been able to make it there every time.

On Thursday, October 23, 2008, at 10:23am Mary's life changed. It started as an ordinary day. She was at school teaching her second class of the day when she was struck with a strong, sudden urge to pee. There were four more minutes until the class was over, so she did her best to hold back the urge. It kept getting more severe with each minute that passed. The minutes felt like hours until the bell finally rang.

Mary wasted no time making her way to the bathroom. You see, she has exactly eight minutes to get to her next class and it takes her two and a half minutes just to get to the bathroom. The halls were filled with kids, which made it more difficult than ever. As she turned the corner, she could see the teacher's lounge, so she picked up her pace. Then it happened. Without any warning, Mary's bladder began to empty. Only this time she was unable to stop it. It poured right through her clothes and onto the floor!

Urgent or Not

Urgency, the intense, immediate need to urinate, can happen to anyone at any time in any place because it does not discriminate. However, how you **react** to the bladder's signal of urgency can make all the difference. Unfortunately, Mary chose the wrong reaction, which led her to lose (empty) her entire bladder. It would have been less embarrassing if this happened to Mary when she was at home as she would not have had the audience she had that dreadful day at school. But then, when is life ever easy?

When urgency causes this level of devastation, your life is forever changed. Every thought, every choice, and every opportunity from then on needs to be heavily weighed. Future decisions will no longer be casually made, whether you are planning a long overdue Caribbean vacation or trying to decide if you should pee before you leave the office. After all, each choice could have very serious consequences.

Although this sudden, severe urgency can cause extreme embarrassment, as in Mary's experience, it can also be very easily controlled. The key lies in your **reaction**. Since it is essential your bladder stays calm in this situation, the worst thing you can do is panic and race to the bathroom. Ironically, this is precisely what most women tend to do.

Autonomic Nervous System and Control

This 'panic' Mary experienced kicks your autonomic nervous system (ANS) into high gear. Simply put, your ANS controls your bladder. Once in high gear, it triggers a 'fight or flight' response.

During this response, your body is preparing to protect itself by either 'fighting' back or taking 'flight' (running). In order for either of these choices to be available to you, your arm and leg muscles need to be prepared. Increased blood flow to them is the answer.

Instantly, your ANS tells your heart to pump faster because your arm and leg muscles need more blood and oxygen in order to respond quickly. It also orders your organs to send any extra blood they have to these same muscles for even more assistance.

Many other pathways inside your body are also affected, making the result **internal chaos**.

Your organs are on hyper-alert, which means your bladder is no longer calm. The more you panic, the more your bladder contracts. This is the reason women leak on the way to the bathroom.

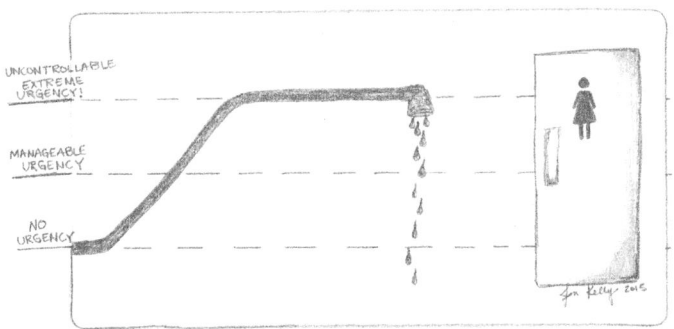

Although she was unaware at the time, if Mary had resisted the impulse to panic, she could have made it to the bathroom without leaking. The best advice in this situation is **do not panic!** When that sudden urge strikes, **STOP** what you are doing immediately.

If you are sitting, do not get up.

If you are standing, do not move.

If you are walking, do not take another step.

Your primary goal *at that moment* is to keep your bladder calm.

In Chapter 2, Test-Taking 101, we learned the bladder should be at rest 99% of the time. Let's take this one level deeper. Picture your autonomic nervous system having two arms. One ANS 'arm' keeps your bladder calm. The other ANS 'arm' allows your bladder to contract.

Chapter 9: Rush Hour

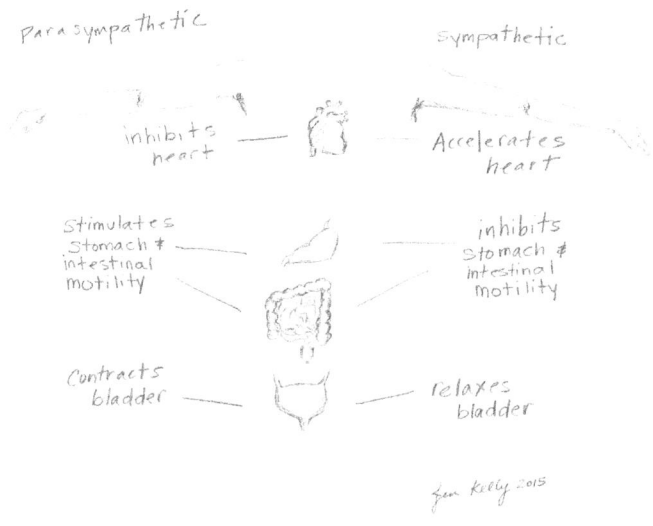

Your bladder should only contract a total of 15 minutes of each day, and only when it is convenient for you to sit on the toilet to pee. For the remaining 23 hours and 45 minutes, the bladder should be calm. In order for this to happen, the 'calm arm' must constantly be on the job. At the same time, the 'contraction arm' hangs in the background just waiting for the chance to make its move.

When you panic, in any situation, the 'contraction arm' takes over. Since both 'arms' cannot work simultaneously, the 'calm arm' must step back. If you allow this 'contraction arm' to stay in control, you will continually leak on the way to the bathroom. It is essential you help the 'calm arm' regain its control so **you must stay calm!**

Try this technique (*The Urgency Technique*) because it works like a charm;

1. Do not panic, or you may begin to leak.
2. For the next five to ten seconds, take a few deep relaxing breaths and say to yourself, "I am not ready, I can do this".

3. Mean what you just said in technique three above and say it again. It is crucial your body and head are in the same place. You cannot think calmly while your body is moving quickly.
4. Once you feel that strong urge begin to dissipate, start walking slowly and calmly to the bathroom.
5. Chant the mantra, "I'm not ready, I can do this" over and again, all the way to the bathroom.
6. Do not stop the mantra when you are unbuttoning your pants or you may start to leak.
7. Once you are sitting on the toilet and ready to pee, you can stop the mantra.

By the way, there is no need to say any of the above out loud unless that is your choice. My guess is you will think the above sounds totally absurd. True, it does sound pretty hokey. However, if you try it, I guarantee you it will work.

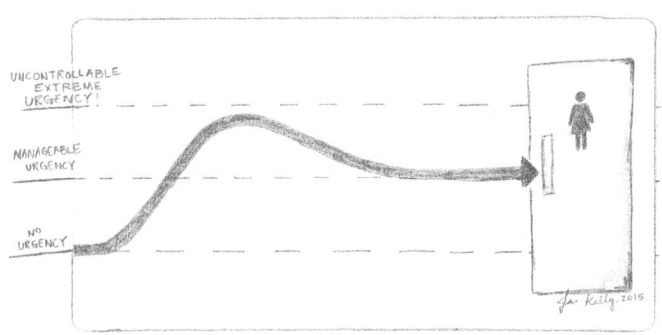

This technique is powerful knowledge. You now have the ability to calm your bladder just enough so you can make it to the bathroom without leaking. And, it can work every time. For those of you who only leak on the way to the bathroom, your days of leaking are over. Hallelujah!

This technique, although fabulous, is only equivalent to placing a huge Band-Aid on your bladder. It will not cure your urgency or leaking, but it will enable you to control it. However, Band-Aids are good, so we'll take it. When you incorporate **all** of the components of my program, only then will you discover the cure. For now, remember — ***mind over bladder**!*

Chapter 10
Bigger Really Is Better

In Chapter 9, Rush Hour, I spoke about the sudden urgent signal to pee and how to calm your bladder so you could make it to the bathroom without leaking. This chapter is about a different type of urge: the normal urge you receive when it is time to pee. Although it, too, may be strong, it is not linked with the feeling of dread about leaking on the way to the bathroom. The severe sudden urgent signal should always be managed as described in Chapter 9, Rush Hour: Stop immediately, think calmly, and tell yourself all the way to the bathroom that you are **not** ready. That said, let's move on to handling the normal, but frequent, urge.

The charts in Chapter 2, Test-Taking 101, are critical to getting women to understand how frequently they pee. This includes middle-aged women who drink coffee in the morning as well as younger mothers who don't take the time to drink anything except at meals.

Maybe there was a day when you got distracted on your way to the bathroom and then forgot you had to pee. Ah, good times. Maybe now, however, you get distracted in the middle of a good movie because you have to pee. My, how times have changed!

If this sounds remotely like you, then your bladder has most likely already shrunk.

Fortunately, this problem can be rectified. Since a muscle can get smaller or shorter, like the hamstrings or your bladder, then it also has the ability to get bigger or longer. A smaller bladder makes you pee more and sleep less. A bigger bladder lets you pee less and sleep more. Therefore, stretching your bladder is the next logical step.

There is a wrong way and a right way to stretch a muscle. I mentioned earlier that my son, Max, broke his arm when he was eight years old. Once the cast was removed, we needed to initiate a stretching program so he could regain the ability to straighten his arm fully. His program involved *comfortably* stretching his arm in a straightened position. We spent about ten minutes of pain-free stretching each session and performed it many times throughout each day until he could finally straighten his arm. This was the right way to stretch a muscle.

The wrong way would have been to force his arm into a straightened position. This would have been uncomfortable for Max and could have caused some muscle injury. Had that been the case, it would have taken even longer for Max to regain all the motion in his arm.

Something I call *The Signal System* is the key to stretching the bladder, similar to the method we used to stretch the muscles on Max's healed arm.

The Signal System

Since not leaking is our goal, we will implement this gentle technique. You will need to work on stretching your bladder throughout each day. Since almost everyone pees first thing in the morning, that is where you will begin. After your first pee of the morning go about your day as usual. Take your shower, have some breakfast, watch the news. Do whatever it is you usually do. At some time, you will get your **first** signal to pee or rather, the first signal since the last time you peed.

At this **first** signal, I want you to acknowledge it and then pick a small project to **distract** yourself. For example, let's say you are reading the newspaper when you get the first signal that you have to pee. Acknowledge it; "Yes, I know I have to pee." Then find something that will take you 10-15 minutes to do and do it; "I'm just going to finish reading this section of the paper and then I'll go to the bathroom."

This is the time when your bladder is allowed to stretch. It is crucial to stay focused on your "project." When you get your

second signal, your reminder signal, walk calmly to the bathroom and pee. Then, start the process all over again. Each **first** signal, distract yourself and each **second** signal, walk calmly to the bathroom and pee.

Do not try to wait until the third signal. Overstretching your bladder is too aggressive and will most likely cause you to leak. And that leak could very well be a large one.

I want you to use this technique all day every day. Sometimes you will only be able to wait ten minutes, and that is ok. Maybe your bladder really was full. Sometimes, however, you will be able to wait an extra hour, which is fantastic! That means your bladder was probably irritated, but you were able to override that feeling so your bladder could continue filling.

Since you now know how to stretch your bladder properly, we need to make sure you always do so. You **must not** pee unless you get a signal to pee. To explain, let's review some bladder facts.

1. The Ferocious Four (caffeine, alcohol, carbonation, and acidic drinks) and the Invisible Irritants (the lack of water or good fluids) are mainly responsible for bladder irritation.
2. An irritated bladder makes the inner walls of the bladder feel itchy and twitchy, making you feel like you need to pee.
3. This need to pee makes you empty your bladder before it is full.
4. Emptying your bladder before it is full on a regular basis leads to bladder shrinkage.
5. Bladder shrinkage leads to nighttime peeing.

Fact 4 above talks about emptying a bladder before it is full. This usually happens because the bladder is irritated, causing the signal to come too soon. There is another reason that is less obvious. Many women believe if they empty their bladder often enough, even when they do not have the urge to pee, they are preventing a leak from happening. Their logic: an empty bladder has nothing in it to leak. They tend to pee every time they leave their houses.

This type of behavior is called peeing "**just in case.**" When you choose to empty your bladder too soon, you are essentially emptying it of not only urine, but of any good fluids you drank as well.

Remember, the good fluids serve to keep the urine **neutral** and calm. If you rid your bladder of these 'neutralizers,' then it begins to fill again with concentrated urine. In addition, you may not drink anything else for some time, which means the urine in your bladder stays concentrated. Concentrated urine is as irritating as a cup of caffeinated coffee!

Peeing "just in case" does not work. There will always be urine in your bladder because the kidneys continuously produce urine. Instead, it contributes to bladder shrinkage and only makes your symptoms worse. You cannot successfully stretch your bladder and shrink it simultaneously. The peeing "just in case" must stop.

Finally, remember to drink your fluids, evenly spaced, throughout each day. These fluids keep the urine diluted and the bladder's environment calm. A calm bladder is easy to stretch. You cannot have success without these fluids on board.

Use *The Signal System* consistently each day to allow your bladder to stretch back to its original size. Once you go to bed, you are done stretching your bladder for the day. There is nothing you can do in the middle of the night to distract yourself. If your bladder wakes you up, get up, pee, and go back to sleep.

As you work on this each day, you will quickly see improvements. In a very short amount of time, you will find you can wait four hours to pee without any difficulty. I have seen this happen in as little as one week. When four hours during the day becomes your norm, you will be sleeping through the night. That's right, I said sleeping through the night in just a few weeks!

Ex. The Signal System
1. First signal–acknowledge it and distract yourself
2. Second signal–calmly go to the bathroom
3. Never pee 'just in case'
4. Drink all your daily fluids evenly spaced

Chapter 11
More Muscles That Matter

Up until now, we have only discussed which techniques need to be implemented to address your 'unstable' bladder. Once your bladder becomes stable, your symptoms should drastically improve. We are not done yet, however.

Your bladder is only one of the very important muscles involved in curing your symptoms. Other muscles of equal importance are the pelvic floor muscles.

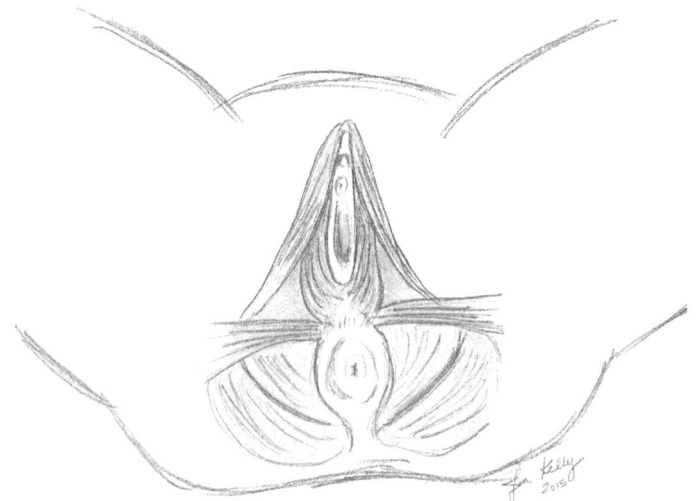

Chapter 11: More Muscles That Matter

As you can see in the diagram, this group of muscles actually lines the floor of the pelvis. The pelvic floor is made up of layers of muscle that collectively perform two very important functions. One function supports the internal organs such as the bladder, uterus, vagina, and rectum. The other function keeps us continent by shutting off the unintentional loss of urine and feces.

Organ Support

The pelvic floor muscles are shaped like a hammock and sit at the base of the pelvis. They attach to both sides of the pelvis (left and right), and their length is very important to their function.

Mary's pelvis measures six inches, spanning from the left to right side of her pelvis. Her pelvic floor muscles measure six inches and they are strong because she has been diligent with her pelvic floor exercises. Her bladder, uterus, vagina, and bowels are sufficiently supported and, therefore, all stay where they belong.

Five years later, Mary has fallen out of her exercise routine. Her pelvic floor muscles are now weaker. Because of the effects of gravity, when the pelvic floor muscles weaken, they get a little longer or sag. If Mary's muscles now measure six and one half inches, for instance, then her organs do not have the full support they did previously. For Mary, this means her organs may be seated a little lower in the pelvis than before.

If these organs continue to drop, or prolapse, lower into the pelvis, any one of them can end up bulging through the vagina, causing pressure, pain, or leaking from the bladder or bowels. Regular exercise of the pelvic floor muscles is needed to prevent these problems from happening.

Flow Control

The bladder is an *involuntary* muscle: you cannot contract it on command. As stated previously the bladder should only contract when it is full and ready to empty. By now, with the techniques you have already learned, you are able to make it to the bathroom before that happens.

The pelvic floor muscles are *voluntary* muscles just like the muscles in your arms and legs. For example, when you decide to take a drink of water (which should be quite often by now) you need to contract the muscles of your hand to hold the glass. Then you need to contract the muscles of your elbow and shoulder to bring the glass to your mouth. You did this without much thought.

The pelvic floor muscles, when working properly, operate the same way. When you laugh, cough, or sneeze, your pelvic floor muscles contract without conscious effort. It is their job to make sure nothing passes that should not pass (i.e., pee, poop, or gas) during these activities.

If you are experiencing any episodes of leaking, your pelvic floor muscles are probably too weak to prevent the pee, poop, or gas from escaping.

Any muscle that is not regularly used becomes weak. We constantly exercise our bigger muscles just by performing everyday activities like bathing, cooking, and walking. These simple activities help prevent those bigger muscles from becoming weak.

Our pelvic floor muscles are not as lucky because they are not used during most daily activities. Let's face it: unless you are specifically exercising the pelvic floor muscles, the only time they get to work out is during intercourse. So, if that is a daily activity for you, your pelvic floor muscles are all set. For the rest of you, however, those muscles need more exercise!

Chapter 12
The Inside Workout

So your pelvic floor muscles probably need more exercise, and the beauty of exercising them is it can be incorporated into your daily routine. You do not have to spend money to join a gym or put aside an extra hour each day in your already busy schedule.

Pelvic floor exercises can be done at the breakfast table or when you are watching your favorite program on television. You can do them standing at the kitchen counter or while you are taking a shower. You can even do them while having intercourse!

These exercises are easy to perform and extremely effective. Regardless of where you choose to do them, there are two important facts you will need to remember.

First, the pelvic floor muscles are small, so they are easily fatigued. Just as pacing is important with your fluids, it is also important with exercising your pelvic floor muscles. If they are not allowed enough time to rest between exercise sets, they will become too fatigued to prevent a leak.

Second, muscles do not get stronger overnight. A muscle needs consistent exercise over several months to gain noticeable strength. I will try to explain this without getting too technical. When a physical therapist tests the strength of a muscle, that muscle is given a 'grade.' The grades range from zero to five with five being 'normal.' Any grade lower than a five means the muscle is weak.

Let's pretend your pelvic floor muscles receive a grade of two out of five. In order to increase that to a grade of three out of five, you would need to exercise them **consistently** and **effectively** for a period of four to six weeks. Therefore, it would take you a total of 12 to 18 weeks of consistent and effective exercise for your pelvic floor muscle strength to be normal, or five out of five.

Thankfully, we do not need our pelvic floor muscles to be a five out of five in order to stop the leaking. We do, however, need to exercise them consistently and effectively to gain enough control to make a difference. And it can happen in as little as a few weeks!

Exercising Your Pelvic Floor Muscles

When I mention pelvic floor exercises to women, most of them think of the Kegel (pronounced 'key-gul') exercise. When performed correctly, the Kegel is an excellent exercise that makes the pelvic floor muscles lift up inside your pelvis toward your bladder. This was the original pelvic floor exercise published by Dr. Arnold Kegel in 1948.

Unfortunately, when your pelvic floor muscles are weak, the effectiveness of the Kegel for pelvic floor strengthening is diminished. I have other exercises I prefer to begin with when this is the case (as it almost always is). Once you have had sufficient practice exercising your pelvic floor muscles, you can begin learning the Kegel.

My two favorite exercises for the pelvic floor muscles are the Roll-In and the Pelvic Brace. Both of these exercises were first described to me during a pelvic floor therapy course I took many years ago taught by Janet Hulme, a physical therapist guru in pelvic floor rehabilitation. The Roll-In exercise is best for long-term strengthening of the pelvic floor muscles and the Pelvic Brace is best for preventing certain types of leaks.

** **Noteworthy**** If you have **ANY** pain in the pelvic floor area, then you should not be performing these exercises. Instead, go see your gynecologist for a consult. Pain in the pelvic region can translate into tight pelvic floor muscles. If your muscles are tight, then the last thing you should do is try to strengthen them because that will cause tighter pelvic floor muscles and more pain.

The Roll-In

The Roll-In is a simple seated exercise that feels like nothing more than an inner thigh exercise. Don't be fooled though. Scientific research proves the Roll-In exercise is effective at producing a pelvic floor muscle contraction.

With the use of biofeedback during many of my physical therapy sessions, I can attest that the pelvic floor muscles do, indeed, produce a stronger contraction than a Kegel contraction *almost* every time. In fact, over the past 14 years, I have only seen three women with a stronger Kegel contraction than a Roll-In contraction. Of course, those women had been doing Kegels consistently and correctly for years.

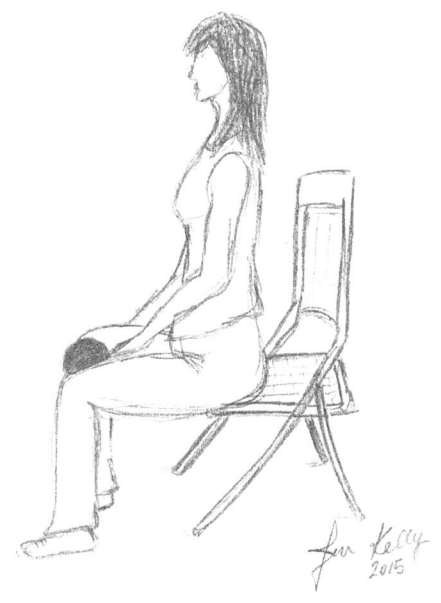

The Roll-In is simple and effective and is performed as follows:

1. Begin by sitting near the edge of a chair that has a firm seat.
2. Sit up straight because good posture is necessary to properly position your pelvic floor muscles for exercise.
3. Place your feet shoulder-width apart and flat on the floor. Use a footstool if the chair is too high for you.
4. Keeping your feet flat on the floor, place a six or seven inch ball (preferred) or pillow between your knees. Firmly squeeze your knees together but do not squeeze them as hard as you can.
5. If you are unable to comfortably squeeze your knees in this position, move your feet a little closer together.
6. Hold this firm squeeze for two normal breaths in and out, which is about 10 seconds.
7. Relax your legs for the next four breaths in and out. (The best way to strengthen a muscle is to make the relax phase twice as long as the contraction phase.)
8. Repeat this squeeze and relax process 10-15 times in one sitting.
9. By the way, now would be a good time to have another glass of water!

** **Noteworthy**** If you have had total hip replacement surgery in the past, please check with your doctor regarding your total hip precautions before performing this exercise.

This simple exercise should be performed between three and five times each day. Some women like to use mealtimes (since they are already sitting) for three of them and then add the other two times between meals. This works well because the exercises are not performed too close together. Remember, these muscles are small, so rest time is as important as exercise time.

The Pelvic Brace

The Pelvic Brace exercise can be performed in any position (lying down, sitting, standing, or moving), but the effects of gravity on the pelvic floor muscles dictate its level of difficulty. Lying down is technically the easiest position for a pelvic floor contraction, but not necessarily the most convenient for you. The seated position is the second easiest position: it's easy to perform, and it's a more convenient position for an exercise.

The Pelvic Brace can be a little challenging at first because it involves 3 simultaneous functions: a Kegel contraction, a transverse abdominal contraction, and active breathing. As with any difficult procedure, we will simplify it into steps.

A Kegel contraction, which we briefly discussed earlier, is important to learn because it plays a special role in the prevention of certain leaks. I like to describe a Kegel in 3 ways:

1. Pretend you are startled by a sudden noise when you are in your bathroom peeing. Your reaction is to stop peeing so you can figure out from where the sound came. The action you use to shut off the flow of urine midstream is a Kegel. This is how you do a Kegel, but *not when* you should do one. Continually trying to stop the flow of urine midstream as an exercise can cause problems with the neurological component of urination.
2. Pretend you are on an elevator with a couple of strangers. Your belly is really bubbly but you do not want to pass gas. You pull in with the muscles surrounding your anus to avoid embarrassment. The action you use to squeeze your anus is also a Kegel.
3. Pretend you are having intercourse and you try to squeeze your partner's penis with the muscles in your vagina. The action you use to squeeze his penis is again a Kegel. Some women use this technique to find out from their partner if their pelvic floor muscles are getting stronger. He is like your own personal biofeedback machine!

Each one of these scenarios is an example of how to perform a Kegel. Since all of your pelvic floor muscles are connected, you cannot contract one without contracting all of them.

Once a woman understands how to perform a Kegel and practices it a few times, I move on to the transverse abdominal exercise. These two exercises are essential for the pelvic brace.

The transverse abdominal muscles are the deepest layer of abdominal muscles, which start at your sides and span across to the center of your belly. They compress and support the organs in the abdominal cavity, including the bladder.

To contract the transverse abdominal muscles, pretend you are putting on a pair of jeans that are a little snug. You need to draw your belly button in toward your spine to allow the zipper to close. The action you use to do this is a transverse abdominal contraction.

Now that you understand how to perform a Kegel contraction and a transverse abdominal contraction, you are ready for the Pelvic Brace. The Pelvic Brace is performed as follows:

1. Begin by sitting near the edge of a chair that has a firm seat.
2. Sit up straight because good posture is necessary to properly position your pelvic floor muscles for exercise.
3. Place your feet flat on the floor. Use a footstool if the chair is too high for you.
4. Make your pelvic floor muscles pull up by performing a Kegel using one of the above three descriptions.
5. Pull your belly in by performing a transverse abdominal contraction.
6. Inhale.
7. Exhale.
8. Relax the pelvic floor and transverse abdominal muscles.

This exercise is particularly challenging because the transverse abdominal muscles connect to the diaphragm, which allows you to breathe. Not only are you trying to do three things at once, which takes much coordination, but you are also limiting the movement of your diaphragm, which makes it more difficult to breathe.

Chapter 12: The Inside Workout

Practice the pelvic brace five to ten times in a row, or until is feels less challenging. As with most things, the more you practice it, the easier it becomes.

Now that you know how to perform a Pelvic Brace, it is time to put it to good use. The Pelvic Brace is one of my favorite exercises because it helps prevent leaks associated with common leak-provoking activities. The most common ones I hear about are leaks associated with coughing, getting up from a chair, getting out of a car, getting out of a bed, and squatting down.

We already discussed the technique to prevent a leak when you have a strong urge, which is to think calmly and walk slowly to the bathroom. This technique, unfortunately, won't do a thing to prevent a leak from a cough. This is because the mechanics behind the leaking are different. A leak with a strong urge, also known as urge incontinence, occurs as the bladder contracts when it should be at rest. A leak with a cough, also known as stress incontinence, is due to the amount of pressure exerted on the bladder during a cough.

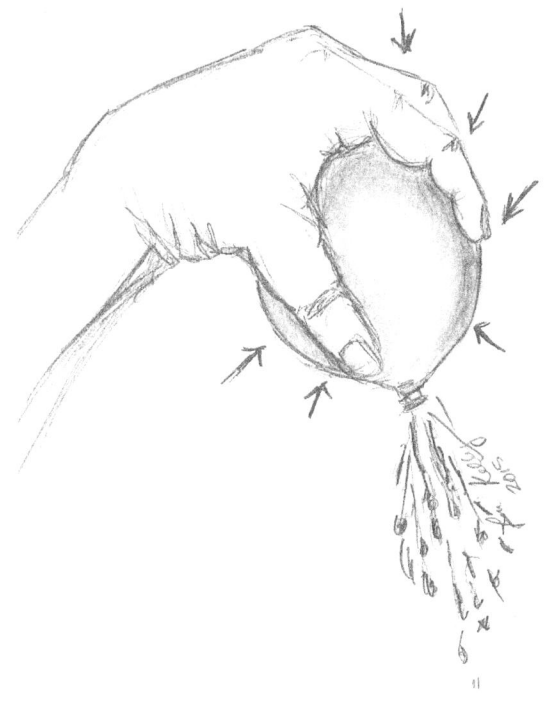

Picture a balloon filled with water. If you exert enough pressure on the balloon, it will burst because there is no other place for the water to go. The same idea applies to the bladder, except the bladder will not burst. The pressure from a cough travels through the abdominal cavity and hits the bladder with a strong force. Since the bladder is not tied closed like the balloon, the urine will get pushed toward the bladder opening, causing a potential leak.

Normally the pelvic floor muscles are strong enough to counter that force by automatically contracting to close off the bladder. The potential leak is avoided and you are none the wiser.

However, if the pelvic floor muscles are weak, they are unable to squeeze hard enough and the result is a leak. This is where the Pelvic Brace exercise comes in handy. Right before you are about to cough, do the Pelvic Brace. And do not let it go until you are done coughing.

Alone, your pelvic floor muscles may not be strong enough to prevent a leak from a cough, but with your help (and the Pelvic Brace) you should be all set.

Use this same technique with every activity that makes you leak. If moving from sitting to standing makes you leak, then do a Pelvic Brace first and hold it throughout the movement. The same goes for getting out of a car and getting out of a bed.

The most common complaint I hear from women about this prevention technique is they forget to use it. When they do use it, however, it works great. To increase the likelihood of performing the Pelvic Brace with the activity that makes you leak, you will need to practice it as an exercise with that activity.

For example, if coughing makes you leak, then your exercise will be as follows:

1. Begin by sitting near the edge of a chair that has a firm seat.
2. Sit up straight because good posture is necessary to properly position your pelvic floor muscles for exercise.
3. Place your feet flat on the floor. Use a footstool if the chair is too high for you.
4. Perform a Pelvic Brace.

5. While holding the Pelvic Brace, cough into your elbow.
6. When done coughing, relax the Pelvic Brace.
7. Repeat this exercise 10 times in a row at least one time a day *and* every time you cough.

By practicing the Pelvic Brace with a cough, you are training your body to remember to use this technique every time you cough. Essentially, you are creating a good habit, and the result will be coughing without leaking.

Any activity can be substituted for the cough. You can practice the Pelvic Brace with getting out of bed if that's what makes you leak. You can practice it with squatting down to pick something up if that's what makes you leak.

Just pay attention to the activities that make you leak and conquer them one by one by turning them into this exercise. Initially, the burden will be on you to remember. Creating a list of which activities to practice with the pelvic brace may be helpful. Eventually, it will involve no thought on your part. It will occur automatically, which is exactly the goal!

CHAPTER 13
WHAT GOES IN MUST COME OUT

Remember Judy? Judy was introduced in Chapter Three as the 44-year old mother of three teenaged children who had problems associated with her bladder.

Let's take a look at Judy's Urinary Incontinence Impact Questionnaire and three day Input & Output Diary to understand why her problems might be happening.

Chapter 13: What Goes In Must Come Out

Urinary Incontinence Impact Questionnaire

Frequency of urinary leaks (small & large):	The longest time I can wait to pee is:
0 I do not leak at all	0 4 hours
1 I leak 1-3 times a month	1 3 1/2 hours
2 I leak 1-3 days a week	2 3 hours
3 I leak 4-6 days a week	3 2 1/2 hours
4 I leak 1-3 times a day	**(4)** 2 hours
5 I leak 3-6 times a day	5 1 1/2 hours
(6) I leak more than 6 times a day	6 1 hour
7 I dribble all day long	7 1/2 hour or less
At most, I wear ___ pads in 24 hours:	**The shortest time I can wait to pee is:**
0 0	0 4 hours
1 1	1 3 1/2 hours
2 2	2 3 hours
3 3	3 2 1/2 hours
4 4	4 2 hours
(5) 5	5 1 1/2 hours
6 6	**(6)** 1 hour
7 More than 6	7 1/2 hour or less
I drink ___ glasses of fluid each day:	**At most, I wake up ___ times at night to pee:**
0 8 or more	0 0
1 7	1 1
2 6	2 2
3 5	3 3
(4) 4	**(4)** 4
5 3	5 5
6 2	6 6
7 Less than 2	7 More than 6
The types of protection I use are:	**I leak with ___. (Circle all that apply)**
0 None	0 N/A
1 Folded tissue paper	**(1)** Cough, sneeze, laugh
(2) Panty liners	1 Sports, exercise, running, jumping
3 Small pads	1 Getting out of bed
4 Medium pads	1 Getting out of a car
5 Large pads	**(1)** Getting up from a chair
6 Two pads at the same time	**(1)** The sound of running water
7 Pull-up style	**(1)** Urgency or trying to get to the bathroom

Date: 5/18/10   Score: 35 /56

At a quick glance, we see that Judy has more than six accidents a day, urinates as often as every hour, and wakes up four times a night to pee. Also, she only drinks 4 fluids a day, which we already know can cause many of her problems.

Now let's look at one of the days Judy recorded during her three-day diary.

The Art Of Control

Input & Output Diary

Date	Time	Fluid Intake	Void in Toilet	Accident	Comments
5/18/10	11:45 pm		M		up at night to pee
5/19/10	1:45 am		M		up at night to pee
	2:20 am		S		up at night to pee
	5:00 am		M		up at night to pee
	7:00 am		S	S	on way to bathroom
	8:10 am	6 oz coffee			with caffeine
	8:15 am		S	M	sneezed
	9:00 am		S	S	on way to bathroom
	10:30 am	6 oz coffee		S	caffeine, stood up from chair
	11:45 am		M		
	1:15 pm		S		
	2:00 pm		S	S	on way to bathroom
	2:15 pm	8 oz milk			
	4:00 pm		M		
	4:30 pm	8 oz water			
	6:00 pm		M		
	7:00 pm		S	S	on way to bathroom
	8:10 pm		S		
	8:45 pm			S	stood up from chair
	9:00 pm		S		
	10:30 pm		S		bedtime

In this particular 24 hours, Judy peed 16 times and had seven accidents.

Take a look at the Fluid Intake column, and you will see Judy drank a total of 36 ounces for the entire day. That is only 50% of the daily fluid her bladder needs to stay calm. Also of note, 16 of those 36 ounces included caffeine, which is one of the Ferocious Four bladder irritants. Now, let me show you what else I see when I look at this diary.

Chapter 13: What Goes In Must Come Out

The first thing I do when analyzing one of these diaries is calculate the amount of time between fluids and group them in circles.

Input & Output Diary

Date	Time	Fluid Intake	Void in Toilet	Accident	Comments
5/18/10	11:45 pm		M		up at night to pee
5/19/10	1:45 am		M		up at night to pee
	2:20 am		S		up at night to pee
	5:00 am		M		up at night to pee
	7:00 am		S	S	on way to bathroom
	8:10 am	6 oz coffee			with caffeine
	8:35 am		S	M	sneezed
	9:00 am		S	S	on way to bathroom
	10:30 am	6 oz coffee		S	caffeine, stood up from chair
	11:45 am		M		
	1:15 pm		S		
	2:00 pm		S	S	on way to bathroom
	2:15 pm	8 oz milk			
	4:00 pm		M		
	4:30 pm	8 oz water			
	6:00 pm		M		
	7:00 pm		S	S	on way to bathroom
	8:10 pm		S		
	8:45 pm			S	stood up from chair
	9:00 pm		S		
	10:30 pm		S		bedtime

Group 1: 2+ hrs. (first fluid group)
Group 2: 3.5 hrs.
Group 3: 2.5 hrs.
Group 4: 6 hrs.

In this case, there is a little more than two hours between the first and second fluids and about three and a half hours between the second and third fluids. There is also two and a half hours between the third and fourth fluids and then six more hours between the fourth fluid and bedtime.

69

Since the Fluid Intake column affects the Void in Toilet column, the next thing I do is group the voids that fall within the same timeframes as the fluid groups.

Now that we have four distinct groups of time, we can begin to see the relationship between the Fluid Intake and Void in Toilet columns as follows:

Input & Output Diary

Date	Time	Fluid Intake	Void in Toilet	Accident	Comments
5/18/10	11:45 pm		M		up at night to pee
5/19/10	1:45 am		M		up at night to pee
	2:20 am		S		up at night to pee
	5:00 am		M		up at night to pee
	7:00 am		S	S	on way to bathroom
	8:30 am	6 oz coffee	2x		with caffeine
	8:35 am		S	M	sneezed
	9:00 am		S	S	on way to bathroom
	10:30 am	6 oz coffee	3x	S	caffeine, stood up from chair
	11:45 am		M		
	1:15 pm		S		
	2:00 pm		S	S	on way to bathroom
	2:15 pm	8 oz milk	1x		
	4:00 pm		M		
	4:30 pm	8 oz water			
	6:00 pm		M 5x		
	7:00 pm		S	S	on way to bathroom
	8:30 pm		S		
	8:45 pm			S	stood up from chair
	9:00 pm		S		
	10:30 pm		S		bedtime

Group 1: 2 hrs.
Group 2: 3.5 hrs.
Group 3: 2.5 hrs.
Group 4: 6 hrs.

Group 1: Judy had six ounces of coffee, with caffeine, during the first two hours. During this same two hours, she peed two times.

CHAPTER 13: WHAT GOES IN MUST COME OUT

Input & Output Diary

Date	Time	Fluid Intake	Void in Toilet	Accident	Comments
	8:30 am	6 oz coffee			with caffeine
	8:45 am		S	M	sneezed
	9:00 am		M	S	on way to the bathroom

Group 2: Judy had six more ounces of coffee, with caffeine, during the next three and a half hours. During this same amount of time, she peed three times.

Input & Output Diary

Date	Time	Fluid Intake	Void in Toilet	Accident	Comments
	10:30 am	6 oz coffee		S	caffeine, stood up from chair
	11:45 am		M		sneezed
	1:15 pm		S		
	2:00 pm		S	S	on way to bathroom

Group 3: Judy drank 16 ounces of good fluids (eight ounces of milk and eight ounces of water) during the next two and a half hours and only peed one time.

Input & Output Diary

Date	Time	Fluid Intake	Void in Toilet	Accident	Comments
	2:15 pm	8 oz milk			
	4:00 pm		M		
	4:30 pm	8 oz water			

Group 4: Judy had nothing else to drink for the rest of the evening. During those last six hours, she peed five more times.

Input & Output Diary

Date	Time	Fluid Intake	Void in Toilet	Accident	Comments
	6:00 pm		M		
	7:00 pm		S	S	on way to bathroom
	8:10 pm		S		
	8:45 pm			S	stood up from chair
	9:00 pm		S		
	10:30 pm		S		bedtime

The above information can be summed up in two statements:

RULE # 1

The less you drink, the more you pee.
The more you drink, the less you pee.

These two statements should sound familiar because they were originally introduced in Chapter 5, You Irritate Me. Remember we are talking about good (non-irritating) fluids. Had Judy consumed more irritating fluids, she would have peed even more.

Finally, I section off the Accident column according to the same timeline to show the relationship between fluid input, fluid output, and leaking.

Here, we see something very interesting by following the same delineation of groups as we did earlier. Judy had accidents during three out of the four groups of time. She leaked three times during the first group, two times during the second group, zero times in the third group, and two times in the fourth group.

In fact, the only time Judy did not leak was when she drank 16 ounces of good fluids over two and a half hours. In other

CHAPTER 13: WHAT GOES IN MUST COME OUT

words, the only time Judy did not leak was when she drank the most amount of fluid in the shortest amount of time!

Input & Output Diary

Date	Time	Fluid Intake	Void in Toilet	Accident	Comments
5/18/10	11:45 pm		M		up at night to pee
5/19/10	1:45 am		M		up at night to pee
	2:20 am		S		up at night to pee
	5:00 am		M		up at night to pee
	7:00 am		S	S	on way to bathroom
	8:10 am	6 oz coffee	2↑	2↑	with caffeine
	8:15 am		S	M	sneezed
	9:00 am		S	S	on way to bathroom
	10:30 am	6 oz coffee	3X	S	caffeine, stood up from chair
	11:45 am		M	2↑	
	1:15 pm		S		
	2:00 pm		S	S	on way to bathroom
	2:15 pm	8 oz milk	1X	∅	
	4:00 pm		M		
	4:30 pm	8 oz water			
	6:00 pm		M 5X	2↑	
	7:00 pm		S	S	on way to bathroom
	8:10 pm		S		
	8:45 pm			S	stood up from chair
	9:00 pm		S		
	10:30 pm		S		bedtime

Group 1 — 2+ hrs. (8:10 am – 9:00 am)
Group 2 — 3.5 hrs. (10:30 am – 2:00 pm)
Group 3 — 2.5 hrs. (2:15 pm – 4:30 pm)
Group 4 — 6 hrs. (6:00 pm – 10:30 pm)

Hence, I will postulate the following regarding *good fluids*:

RULE # 2

The less you drink, the more you leak.
The more you drink, the less you leak.

This is exactly what happened to Judy. She only drank four fluids all day long, two of which irritated her bladder. She assumed if she drank less, then she would not only pee less, but leak less as well. Unfortunately, she had it all wrong.

Chapter 14
The Medication Fixation & Surgery Surge

"Does that bladder medication work for you?"
"I'm not really sure but I'm afraid to stop taking it in case it really does."
That answer never ceases to amaze me! I understand it, of course, but how sad is that?

Medication

I have treated thousands of women with bladder symptoms, and most of those women had either already tried some type of bladder medication or were still taking one when they came to see me.

Now, I'm a firm believer in medicine when it is warranted. But, when **is** bladder urgency or incontinence medication necessary? If you ask me, the answer would be 'almost never.'

In the past 14 years, I have only had **one** woman who had difficulty weaning off her bladder medication because of increased bladder symptoms. I just worked that much harder to impress upon her the importance of the intricacies of fluid intake and output on her bladder problems. Eventually, she was able to wean off her bladder medication without any adverse bladder affects. I'm a Taurus, and Stubborn is my middle name!

For years, I have tried to educate physicians about the efficacy of physical therapy for treating bladder and bowel symptoms instead of using a medication as their first line of defense. It is unfortunate that I have only a few dozen doctors who understand how powerful physical therapy treatments are in treating urinary symptoms, because there are so many more who do not. The ones who do, however, are now firm believers, and for that I am grateful.

My biggest advocates over the years have been the women I have treated. You see, they tell a friend about their great results with physical therapy, who tells another friend, and so on, and so on. Before I know it, new referrals are coming in from doctors who have never referred to me before, and it is because their patients are requesting it! I can't begin to tell you how great that is. Gone are the days when women keep silent!

As you can see, bladder medications are not the answer. What they do is mask the real problem, and not very well from what I have seen. In addition, they cause all sorts of side effects we certainly do not need.

So for all of you who are currently using bladder medications, there is hope for you to stop taking them and still get rid of your bladder symptoms. Imagine how much healthier your body will be without those chemicals, not to mention how much fatter your pocketbook will grow.

For peace of mind, however, do not stop your bladder medications until you have a) seen good results with the techniques we have discussed and b) run it by your doctor just to be safe. There is no need to try to stop them if you are just starting my program. If anything, it would probably stress you out causing worsening bladder symptoms.

When you *are* ready to try, though, the best way to stop medication is to wean off of it. For example, if you take one pill a day, then wean down to one pill every other day for at least one to two weeks. Next, wean down to one pill every third day for another one to two weeks. Then you can stop taking them all together. I am by no means an expert on weaning off of medications, so make sure you confirm with your doctor or pharmacist the proper way to do so before you begin.

Chapter 14: The Medication Fixation & Surgery Surge

Surgery

The rise in bladder surgeries is astronomical. Between 1979 and 2004, the number of bladder surgeries for incontinence in women more than doubled. Today, more than 100,000 of these surgeries are performed on women each year. My question to you is this: are all of those surgeries necessary?

I have been treating women with bladder prolapses for many years, and I am here to tell you most of the women I treated who were trying to avoid surgery were successful!

If a prolapse is either severe enough to see externally with a mirror or is very painful, it may need to be treated with surgery. Even with the surgery, physical therapy is necessary to prevent further problems.

One time, a urologist shook my hand and thanked me for 'curing' his patients despite the fact it lessened the number of surgeries he was able to perform. He actually said that. It was awesome! To this day, he still sends me his patients despite the fact that I don't even treat in his town anymore. Thank God for the physicians who prefer to treat their patients with the least invasive, non-pharmaceutical treatment possible!

It is also my belief that physical therapy should always be your first treatment choice for organ prolapse. It amazes me how some women can't be bothered to try physical therapy. I know this because I have seen it first hand.

I have a great relationship with a local OBGYN office that requires all of its prolapse surgery candidates to try physical therapy first. That is so cool! Of all the women *required* by them to see me, I have had two who have told me they were just 'going through the motions' so they could have surgery. That breaks my heart. How can some women be so callous with their bodies?

I wonder if those two women knew of all the things that could go wrong with surgery. The list of complications is long. Let's take a look at what can happen:

1. Trouble urinating
2. Permanent urinary retention (unable to fully empty the bladder without possible intermittent catheterization)

3. Abscess
4. Bladder spasms
5. Bleeding
6. Blood clots
7. Injury to the bladder, urethra, and other urinary tract structures
8. Infection (catheter-related infections are the most common)
9. Overactive bladder
10. Reactions to anesthesia
11. Vaginal prolapse
12. Infection or reduced effectiveness of man-made sling material that may wear away
    a. Reactions to anesthesia
    b. Painful intercourse

I can't imagine taking all those risks for an unnecessary surgery. And did I mention that it doesn't always eliminate the leaking or stop at just one surgery? I have met many women who have had bladder surgery two and three times and, yes; they were still referred to me for incontinence!

So, before you decide to take medications or to go 'under the knife,' please try my techniques. They really do work!

Chapter 15
Do As I Say <u>And</u> As I Do

Every woman I work with has a home program designed specifically for her. Her symptoms and feedback drive my treatment plan. Since I do not have *your* feedback to help me design your program, I have designed this general home program, which will definitely do the trick.

The more closely you follow this program, the better your results. Remember, timing is of the essence when it comes to your fluid intake. If it seems I am picky, then I have done my job!

While your bladder is still unstable, it, too, is very picky. So, it is essential you space your fluids as closely as this program recommends. When you do, you will be amazed at how quickly you notice results.

For those of you who do not drink enough fluid each day and are afraid to start, do not fear. You *might* have to pee a little more frequently at first, but only for the first day or two. My guess, however, is you will notice no increase in voiding frequency at all. Remember what we learned in Chapter 11, More Muscles That Matter: the **more** we drink, the **less** we pee!

Good luck to you and your bladder!

Comprehensive Home Program

A. Fluid Intake Schedule

Your first drink starts as soon as you get up for the day. I will use 6:00 A.M. as our example. If you get up at a different time, adjust this schedule accordingly.

6:00 A.M.	8 ounces of water then 8 ounces of coffee (coffee if you wish, with or without caffeine)
8:00 A.M.	8 ounces of water or good fluid
10:00 A.M.	8 ounces of water or good fluid
12:00 P.M.	8 ounces of water or good fluid
2:00 P.M.	8 ounces of water or good fluid
4:00 P.M.	8 ounces of water or good fluid
6:00 P.M.	8 ounces of water or good fluid
8:00 P.M.	8 ounces of water or good fluid

This schedule ensures you drink at least eight ounces of fluid every two hours, which is the longest amount of time between drinks you should allow. Optimally, you should drink eight ounces every one and a half to two hours but it is fine to start with this slightly more conservative schedule.

Should you feel thirsty between scheduled fluids, please, feel free to quench your thirst. If your body wants fluid, so does your bladder.

B. Bladder Urgency

How we react to that suddenly, strong, urgent signal to urinate can either *make it* or *break it* when it comes to a leak. Remember, if you panic and rush to the bathroom, you will probably leak.

Chapter 15: Do As I Say And As I Do

1. Stop and be still for a few seconds (***THIS IS A MUST***)
2. Take a deep, calming breath in and out.
3. Tell yourself, "I'm not ready, I can do this."
4. Once the urgency starts to dissipate, walk slowly and calmly to the bathroom.
5. Tell yourself "I'm not ready" all the way to the bathroom until you are sitting on the toilet.
6. Be free — pee!

It is imperative that your mind and body are in sync during this technique. It is impossible for your brain to stay calm if your body is still rushing to get to the bathroom. If you can't stay calm, then this technique will not work.

Trust your body. You will be amazed how much control you actually have over your bladder.

C. Fluid Output Schedule

The key points to remember about peeing are:

1. Do not pee on the first bladder signal; wait until the second signal.
2. Do not wait past the second signal to pee or you may leak.
3. Do not pee 'just in case.' If you do not have the signal to pee, then don't pee.

D. Exercise

The pelvic floor muscles need exercise. Remember, they have two jobs; one is to support the internal organs of the pelvis, and the other is to stop pee, poop, and gas from leaving the body at inopportune moments.

1. Perform the **Roll-In** exercise three to five times a day, doing 10-15 repetitions each time. Be sure to spread them out throughout the day. The pelvic floor muscles are small and fatigue quickly.

2. Perform the **Pelvic Brace** at least once a day. Practice it with the cough if you leak when you cough. Or, practice it with any other activity that makes you leak like standing up from a chair, getting out of your car, getting up from your bed, etc.

Perform these exercises daily. It will ensure your pelvic floor muscles, like your bladder, pull their fair share of the load.

The above four steps, labeled A through D, need to be performed every day to see good results. When these steps are followed, you will certainly notice less peeing and less leaking within the first week of this program. Some women even begin sleeping longer periods at night in that same time frame.

The possibilities are endless. Enjoy your new life!

Chapter 16
FAQs & Tricks of the Trade

I have been drinking three cups of coffee for the past 20 years. Why is it, all of a sudden, the coffee now irritates my bladder?

Picture our bladders working extra hard for years trying to neutralize all of the irritants we have been giving them (for example, caffeine, soda, alcohol, acidic drinks, and the invisible irritant).

Imagine one day our bladders get super tired. Consider them overworked and underpaid. That is the day they throw their proverbial hands up in the air and say, "We're done. We can't do it anymore. It's your problem now!"

You see, it is not all of a sudden, but rather a gradual process that has been sneaking up on us for years. That all-of-a-sudden-day just happens to be the day we start listening to our bodies and take notice.

<u>Trick of the Trade</u>: You can still have three cups of coffee if you just cut down on the caffeine. For example, if you make each coffee with 1/3 caffeine and 2/3 decaf, then those three cups of coffee are like having just one cup as far as the bladder is concerned.

Will I have to do this for the rest of my life?

Taking care of your bladder and pelvic floor muscles is an ongoing process. Look at it this way. Let's say you work really hard to stabilize your weight and finally achieve your goal. Is it then ok to resort back to your old habits? No, but an occasional deviation from your new protocol will not cause an overall problem.

The good news is this: stabilizing your weight can take months or even years while stabilizing your bladder can take only days or weeks.

I have been doing Kegels for years, and it doesn't seem to help. Why is that?

I have two answers for this:

1. That is because more than just your pelvic floor muscles are involved in bladder leakage, which is why I address the bladder and bowels in addition to the pelvic floor muscles. Addressing the bladder first (fluid input and output) will give you the quickest results.
2. Pelvic floor muscles are very small, which makes them particularly difficult to contract effectively. When weak, they are very difficult to isolate during exercise.

To be effective, the Kegel needs strong pelvic floor muscles. To develop strong pelvic floor muscles, start with the Roll-In exercise. Once the pelvic floor muscles become stronger, you can transition to the Kegel.

I only leak on the way to the bathroom. How do I fix that?

You should be using *The Urgency Technique* from Chapter 7, The Constipation Revelation. It can stop your leaks immediately (yes, that means as soon as today). Make sure your brain and your body are on the same page. If you are thinking 'be calm,' then your body must be acting 'calm.'

This is just a *Band-Aid* technique, however, meaning it will not solve the problem of why you leak. To solve that problem, you must follow the entire program. Only then will the urgent signals triggering the leaks stop.

CHAPTER 16: FAQs & TRICKS OF THE TRADE

Why do I leak when I stand up from my chair?

This question has an easy answer. Most people forget to scoot to the edge of their seat before standing up. It is all about using proper body mechanics.

Trying to stand up when your bottom is all the way at the back of the seat (which is where it should be for a good seated posture) throws off your center of gravity. In other words, you have to lean so far forward just to get your balance before you can rise. When you lean that far forward, you physically squash your bladder causing it to leak.

Since it takes more effort from that position, most people end up holding their breath and bearing down when they do stand (like straining to have a bowel movement). All that pressure pushing down squashes the bladder and causes it to leak.

Trick of the Trade: Practice the pelvic brace technique *as an exercise* when you move from sitting to standing. Use the following steps:

1. Scoot to the edge of the seat.
2. Perform the pelvic brace.
3. Stand up.
4. Relax the pelvic brace.
5. Repeat five to ten times in a row each day.

Doing this as an exercise will help train your body to perform the pelvic brace automatically every time you move from sitting to standing. It creates that good habit that helps to prevent a leak.

My bladder empties when I am sleeping. Is there a way I can fix that?

Yes, you absolutely can fix that! Begin by fixing your daytime problems. You may not be leaking in the daytime, but I certainly bet you are peeing way too frequently.

The voiding frequency goal is to pee four hours apart. The reason is this: your bladder takes twice as long to fill during sleep.

If you pee less than four hours apart on a regular basis during the day, then your bladder will have to empty sometime in the middle of the night. When you sleep, everything slows down, including the production of urine. If it takes four hours to fill (meaning before it needs to empty) during the daytime, then it takes eight hours to fill during the night.

If you are one of the unlucky ones, you will sleep through the signal and wake up wet. Otherwise, the signal will wake you up, and you will have to get up to pee.

Once this problem is corrected in the daytime, your bladder will automatically adjust so nighttime will no longer be an issue.

<u>Trick of the Trade</u>: Make sure you space your fluids out evenly throughout the day and drink up until at least two hours before bedtime. If most of your fluids are consumed during the first half of your day, then by the time you go to bed, your bladder will already be irritated. That causes your bladder to wake you during the night.

I leak as I am getting out of bed. Is that normal?

No, that is not normal, but it certainly is common. This one is resolved, again, by using good body mechanics.

Most people try to get out of bed by jack-knifing their bodies instead of log rolling. Jack-knifing, which is similar to a partial sit-up, ends up squashing your bladder causing you to leak. Or, maybe it happens when you try to stand up from the edge of the bed before scooting your bottom forward first, just like when you stand up from a chair.

You can avoid the leak by performing a log roll when getting out of bed. A log roll is when you pretend your body is as straight as a log while you roll onto your side toward the edge of the bed. Once there, use your arms to push you up to a sitting position as you drop your legs off the edge of the bed. The weight of your legs helps to leverage yourself into that sitting position. Once sitting, don't forget to scoot to the edge of the bed before standing up.

<u>Trick of the Trade</u>: Practice the pelvic brace technique *as an exercise* when you get out of bed. Use the following steps;

1. Perform the pelvic brace.
2. Log roll onto your side toward the edge of the bed.
3. Push up with your arms as you drop your legs off the edge of the bed while you are still holding the pelvic brace.
4. Continue to hold the pelvic brace (or perform another one) as you scoot to the edge of the bed.
5. Stand up from the edge of the bed.
6. Relax the pelvic brace.
7. Repeat five to ten times in a row each day.

Doing this as an exercise will help train your body to perform the pelvic brace automatically every time you get out of bed. It creates that good habit that helps to prevent a leak.

I pee so much during the day because I take diuretics. I can't just stop taking them, so what should I do?

The diuretic effects on your bladder only last a few hours from the time you take it. After that timeframe, you can spread out the time between voids just as well as everyone else.

Many of the women I see take diuretics too, and they still get great results with my program.

Can I drink at bedtime if I'm thirsty?

If you feel thirsty, it is your body's way of telling you it needs fluid. Don't ignore it because if your body wants it, then surely you bladder does too. There is nothing wrong with drinking a *good fluid* before bedtime. That is not the reason you get up at night to pee. Just remember to space the rest of your fluids well throughout the day.

Trick of the Trade: Most nights I drink a full glass of water at bedtime because I know it will help the urine in my bladder stay diluted while I sleep. And, I do not get up at night to pee.

How can I remember to drink fluids if I am not thirsty?

Thirst is a physiological drive to our body's need for fluid. As babies, we know when we are hungry and thirsty because our bodies regulate that need. Once quenched, the feeling of thirst dissipates.

Unfortunately, some of us no longer feel thirsty because, too many times, we have ignored that feeling in the past.

For example, our body tells us time and time again when it needs fluids. If we ignore the reminder time and time again, our body accepts the reminders as futile attempts and stops letting us know when it needs fluids. This is why it becomes very difficult to remember to drink fluids.

Our only recourse is to create a thirst. We do this by giving our bodies regularly scheduled fluids throughout each day for a few weeks. The body then becomes accustomed to receiving fluids regularly again. After that period, if you forget or are unable to drink fluids at your scheduled time, your body then takes over and reminds you of your thirst.

The burden, however, then becomes yours to remember to drink your fluids.

Trick of the Trade: Creating a habit takes time and perseverance. Use whatever technique is available to remind you to drink your fluids. Some tricks that are helpful include:

1. Set a kitchen timer to remember
2. Set a cell phone reminder
3. Leave a water bottle at the kitchen sink or on your desk as a visual reminder
4. Keep Dixie cups in the bathrooms so you can take a drink after you pee
5. Leave water bottles in your mudroom so you can grab one or two on your way out the door
6. Leave a water bottle with your car keys
7. Keep a cooler of water in your car where it is easily accessible when you are driving
8. Keep a water bottle on your bedside table
9. Fill a pitcher of water to leave on your kitchen counter

CHAPTER 16: FAQS & TRICKS OF THE TRADE

I was doing so well on your program until just the other day, and now my symptoms seem to be getting worse. Did I do something wrong?

Sometimes life just gets in the way. Occasionally your overall muscle strength is affected by everyday life. Here are three common examples of when your pelvic floor muscles can cause an increase in your bladder symptoms:

1. Menstruation can cause increased bladder symptoms. Estrogen is at its lowest during menstruation. Since muscles need estrogen to be strong, the week during your menstrual cycle is when your pelvic floor muscles will be at their weakest. Estrogen begins dropping the week before your cycle, so it is during that two-week period when you may notice increased accidents.

Once your pelvic floor muscles are strong enough, the menstrual cycle will bear no ill effect in your symptoms. Until then, however, it is not uncommon to notice more leaks during those 14 days.

2. Illness can cause increased bladder symptoms. When you feel under the weather, your whole body is affected. It can cause overall muscle fatigue, including your pelvic floor muscles. Sometimes it feels like you are practicing for a marathon just getting off the couch for a glass of water when you are sick. Think about the size of your arm and leg muscles compared to your pelvic floor muscles. If your very large leg muscles are pooped when you are sick, then so are your very small pelvic floor muscles.

Unfortunately, your pelvic floor muscles are already weak, which is part of the cause of your bladder leakage. Add to that how pooped they feel when you are sick, and your symptoms will probably be worse. As if that isn't bad enough, you may be one of the unlucky ones who also has a nasty cough with your illness. If coughing is one of your triggers for leaking, you will probably leak more during your illness as well.

3. Fatigue and exhaustion can cause increased bladder symptoms. When your body is physically fatigued or exhausted, your muscles are too. Since your pelvic floor muscles are so small compared to your other muscles (arms, legs, trunk), they will

be even weaker than usual and potentially cause more bladder accidents.

Trick of the Trade: Although pads are not the ultimate solution to leakage, they certainly have their place in our world. You may want to wear a pad and carry extras during your menstrual cycle, a time of illness, or a time of fatigue/exhaustion for added protection. Unfortunately, until your muscles are strong enough to overcome the above three situations, this is your best defense.

My problem isn't that I leak; it's that I pee too frequently. Will this program still work for me?

Yes, it will. Frequent urination is also a type of bladder dysfunction. My program begins with stabilizing the bladder. If fluid into the bladder and fluid out of the bladder are not stabilized, your symptoms will get worse. It is just a matter of time. The natural progression of frequent urination is urinary leakage, otherwise known as urinary incontinence.

Does this mean I can never have something to drink that is irritating to my bladder again?

No, it does not. The initial period of bladder stabilization is very important. During this time, you need to limit or eliminate the amount of irritants in your bladder. Once the initial stabilization phase has been reached, your bladder is again able to handle a few irritants without causing bladder symptoms.

This means you have the power over your bladder. If you are going to have a special day and don't want to chance a leak, watch what you drink.

Trick of the Trade: One trick is to drink a glass of water before you drink an irritant. For example, drink a glass of water before your glass of wine. The water will dilute the irritation caused by the wine and cause fewer symptoms.

Another trick is to change your coffee from full caffeine to half caffeine and half decaf. By the time the coffee hits your bladder, it will be 50% less irritating which will cause fewer symptoms.

I keep forgetting to do my exercises. Is there anything I can do to help me remember them?

Creating a habit is effort. One way to remind yourself is to set a timer in your kitchen or on your phone. When the timer sounds, it is time to do some exercises.

Another way is to connect the exercise to an activity. For example, when you sit down to eat a meal, do your roll-ins at the same time. Or, when you stop at a red light or stop sign, do pelvic brace exercises.

Visual cues can also be helpful. Try placing a sticker (like a smiley face) on your bookmark, computer screen, or bathroom mirror. When you see the sticker, do your exercises.

Eventually, you will remember to do the exercises without all the reminders. Until then, use whatever technique you can think of to get your exercises done.

I did a ton of the Roll-Ins and Pelvic Brace exercises this past week, but now I am leaking more than before. Does that make sense?

It makes a lot of sense. Since your pelvic floor muscles are small, they will fatigue more quickly than the bigger muscles of your body.

Therefore, if you do too many pelvic floor exercises (like five hundred or a thousand — yes I have heard of this happening), then your pelvic floor muscles become so fatigued that you leak more. Remember, there is such a thing as too many exercises.

I think I am ready to start weaning off my bladder medications, but I am nervous that my symptoms will get worse. Do you have any suggestions?

Discuss it with your doctor to make sure she agrees on your timing and to get her advice on the proper weaning technique.

I am all for weaning off medication, but some medications can have a backlash effect if weaning is not done properly. Doctors are the experts on medications. I firmly believe any time to wean is a good time as long as you feel ready.

<u>Trick of the Trade</u>: Anxiety can increase bladder symptoms. A good rule of thumb is that bladders take on our emotions. If we are anxious, our bladders are anxious. If we are nervous, our bladders are nervous. If we are calm, our bladders are calm.

If you are nervous about weaning off your medications, now is not the time to try it.

I want to stop wearing pads, but I am afraid. Should I keep wearing them just in case?

If you are ready to wean off of pads, the best place to start is at your house. Wait until you are planning on being home for the day. That way, should you have an accident, the embarrassment is kept to a minimum, and you have a change of clothes right around the corner.

If you decide to try it outside of your home, make sure you are extra careful with your fluids. Remember, improper fluid amount, type, and timing can lead to bladder accidents.

I have been told time and time again that if I lose weight my bladder issues will improve. Will my weight prevent me from seeing results with your program?

Absolutely not! Although losing weight is clinically proven to help with bladder control, it is not the only solution. If it were that easy to lose weight we would all be doing it. I have helped thousands of women overcome bladder issues regardless of their weight.

I can't seem to regulate my bowels. Is there anything over-the-counter that may help me?

I am a big proponent of Miralax. It has been a staple in our house for at least the past five years. It is a great, mild laxative and can be used long term, per our family gastroenterologist. It is now sold over-the-counter in places like Walmart, Rite Aid, and BJ's Wholesale Club.

If you prefer a more natural alternative, prunes can help. We also use a 'special juice' mixture of 50% prune juice and 50% grape juice (since our kids would not eat prunes). The grape cuts the prune flavor and our kids love it. Sometimes, however, it just does not do the trick. What can I say? Genetics aren't always a good thing!

Another good alternative is magnesium. Go to your local health food store and ask about it.

If you have never sought medical attention for your bowels, it is highly recommended you do so.

I keep trying the Urgency Technique when I get a sudden, strong urge to pee, but it isn't working. What am I doing wrong?

My guess is your body is not in sync with your brain. You must stop *everything* you are doing and *be still* before proceeding to the bathroom. You must tell yourself, and mean it, "I am not ready. I can do this." If your body is still semi-quickly proceeding toward the bathroom, then it will not work. Calm is calm is calm.

The autonomic nervous system needs a 100% calm response from both your brain and your body to overcome the bladder contractions that cause the leakage.

I have completed your program but only had minimal improvements. Did I do something wrong?

Unfortunately, some people have more complicated reasons for their bladder issues. When I am treating someone who is not progressing as quickly as I would like, then I will refer to the appropriate medical provider (i.e., urologist, gynecologist, gastroenterologist, etc.). It is time to seek medical advice.

Chapter 17
Diary of a Wimpy Bladder

Remember Judy? She was the 44-year-old mother of three we met in Chapter 3, Muscle Power, who was suffering from urge incontinence. Judy came to me to learn how to fix her problem. On Judy's first session, I gathered as much information as I could about her typical day. As I suspected, Judy lives a crazy life (as do most women). She drinks too many irritants and too few fluids. She is always running from point A to point B, taking care of everyone before herself. She frequently peed and leaked several times each day and got up to pee several times each night. Fortunately, she decided to address her bladder issues before they could progress. And, believe me, they *definitely* would have gotten worse.

It took only three sessions for Judy to learn the important information and obtain her personalized home program: a fluid intake schedule, a bladder schedule, and an exercise schedule.

Judy's Fluid Intake Schedule

She woke up for the day at 5:30 A.M. each morning and was in bed by 10:00 P.M. each night. Her fluid intake schedule had her drinking six to eight ounces of water (or good fluid) every one and a half hours beginning at 6:00 A.M.

She cut back to two cups of coffee in the morning but since half of each cup was decaffeinated coffee, it was the same as having only one cup of an irritant instead of two. Remember, *decaffeinated coffee is not an irritant.* These small changes made a big difference in her symptoms of frequent peeing and leaking, which both declined dramatically.

If she decided to have a glass of wine at night, which she occasionally enjoyed, then she was instructed to have a glass of water first. This way the wine was less irritating once it entered the bladder.

Judy's Bladder Schedule

As instructed, Judy immediately stopped peeing 'just in case.' She was nervous at first but quickly found it was much easier than she had initially anticipated. It did not make her leak more — her big fear.

She incorporated the first signal/second signal technique as well. At the first non-urgent signal to void, she was successfully able to distract herself on many occasions, allowing an extra hour to pass before she had to pee. She peed less frequently and larger amounts of urine each time.

She also remembered to respond with calmness when she was surprised by the urgent signal to pee. What really surprised her, however, was that the urgent signals were now few and far between. Her increased fluid intake was the key.

Now, if she ever happened to get a strong urgent signal, she knew it was because her fluid intake was low. *And,* she knew how to respond to it to prevent a leak.

Lastly, if she was thirsty at bedtime, she had a glass of water. She was no longer concerned that it would wake her up at night to pee. Actually, she was now sleeping better than she had in years because she was no longer getting up three or four times a night to pee.

Judy's Exercise Schedule

Judy began her pelvic floor exercise with the Roll-In exercise. It was so simple to do, required no equipment, and could be done anytime she was sitting down. She decided to incorporate them at mealtime. Since she ate three meals a day while sitting, it was a no-brainer!

She performed 15 repetitions at each sitting, remembering to hold each Roll-In for two full breaths in and out. If she remembered to do some at other times during her day, she considered those bonus exercises. Her goal, however, was to do them three times a day.

Since Judy also leaked with a cough, we added the Pelvic Brace exercise with a cough to be performed ten times in a row each day. This created a habit, allowing her to remember to do the Pelvic Brace each time she coughed, to prevent leaks with coughing.

Judy was amazed how easy her program was to follow and how quickly she saw results. She told me, as most women do, the most difficult part of the program was *remembering* to drink her fluids. She used her iPhone to set up reminders, and it worked brilliantly!

When Judy came to me, she was already scheduled to have bladder suspension surgery six weeks later. She did so well with my program, she happily cancelled the surgery.

Turn the page to see Judy's post-test results.

Chapter 18
Test-Taking 102

Here we are again. Judy completed her program and had excellent results. I educated her about how the bladder works, how fluids affect it, and how specific exercises can help. She followed my advice and implemented all of the strategies I taught her. On her third session with me, I had her fill out another Urinary Incontinence Impact Questionnaire. It is always so amazing to see the results in black and white, *and* she was thrilled with her results!

Remember, Judy's Pre-test looked like this:

Urinary Incontinence Impact Questionnaire

Frequency of urinary leaks (small & large): 0 I do not leak at all 1 I leak 1-3 times a month 2 I leak 1-3 days a week 3 I leak 4-6 days a week 4 I leak 1-3 times a day 5 I leak 3-6 times a day **(6)** I leak more than 6 times a day 7 I dribble all day long	The longest time I can wait to pee is: 0 4 hours 1 3 1/2 hours 2 3 hours 3 2 1/2 hours **(4)** 2 hours 5 1 1/2 hours 6 1 hour 7 1/2 hour or less
At most, I wear ____ pads in 24 hours: 0 0 1 1 2 2 3 3 4 4 **(5)** 5 6 6 7 More than 6	The shortest time I can wait to pee is: 0 4 hours 1 3 1/2 hours 2 3 hours 3 2 1/2 hours 4 2 hours 5 1 1/2 hours **(6)** 1 hour 7 1/2 hour or less
I drink ____ glasses of fluid each day: 0 8 or more 1 7 2 6 3 5 **(4)** 4 5 3 6 2 7 Less than 2	At most, I wake up ___ times at night to pee: 0 0 1 1 2 2 3 3 **(4)** 4 5 5 6 6 7 More than 6
The types of protection I use are: 0 None 1 Folded tissue paper **(2)** Panty liners 3 Small pads 4 Medium pads 5 Large pads 6 Two pads at the same time 7 Pull-up style	I leak with ____. (Circle all that apply) 0 N/A **(1)** Cough, sneeze, laugh 1 Sports, exercise, running, jumping 1 Getting out of bed 1 Getting out of a car **(1)** Getting up from a chair **(1)** The sound of running water **(1)** Urgency or trying to get to the bathroom

Date: 5/18/10   Score: 35 /56

And, her post-test looked like this:

Urinary Incontinence Impact Questionnaire

Frequency of urinary leaks (small & large):	The longest time I can wait to pee is:
(0) I do not leak at all	(0) 4 hours
1 I leak 1-3 times a month	1 3 1/2 hours
2 I leak 1-3 days a week	2 3 hours
3 I leak 4-6 days a week	3 2 1/2 hours
4 I leak 1-3 times a day	4 2 hours
5 I leak 3-6 times a day	5 1 1/2 hours
6 I leak more than 6 times a day	6 1 hour
7 I dribble all day long	7 1/2 hour or less
At most, I wear ___ pads in 24 hours:	The shortest time I can wait to pee is:
(0) 0	0 4 hours
1 1	(1) 3 1/2 hours
2 2	2 3 hours
3 3	3 2 1/2 hours
4 4	4 2 hours
5 5	5 1 1/2 hours
6 6	6 1 hour
7 More than 6	7 1/2 hour or less
I drink ___ glasses of fluid each day:	At most, I wake up ___ times at night to pee:
(0) 8 or more	(0) 0
1 7	1 1
2 6	2 2
3 5	3 3
4 4	4 4
5 3	5 5
6 2	6 6
7 Less than 2	7 More than 6
The types of protection I use are:	I leak with ___. (Circle all that apply)
(0) None	(0) N/A
1 Folded tissue paper	1 Cough, sneeze, laugh
2 Panty liners	1 Sports, exercise, running, jumping
3 Small pads	1 Getting out of bed
4 Medium pads	1 Getting out of a car
5 Large pads	1 Getting up from a chair
6 Two pads at the same time	1 The sound of running water
7 Pull-up style	1 Urgency or trying to get to the bathroom

Date: 6/15/10   Score: 1 /56

As you can see, Judy did great. In 29 days, she was cured of leaking. And, she was full of energy. She now drinks at least eight glasses of good fluids, spread out evenly, and performs her pelvic floor exercises daily. She is able to wait at least three and one half hours between voids, she is sleeping through the night, and she no longer has to wear pads. Judy got her life back in only 29 days!

Now look at the forms you filled out and see if you can see any of the same patterns I just pointed out on Judy's forms. Although not all forms are this clear cut, chances are you will find many similarities.

Implement my techniques and watch your symptoms disappear. Drink more to pee and leak less, and do your exercises. It is that simple. I know you can do it!

Congratulations!

You now have the knowledge necessary to eliminate successfully and prevent bladder accidents. It is very important to remember that no single part of this program will solve all of your bladder problems. By working on just one component, you may improve your symptoms, but you will not be cured. You must address both the bladder and the pelvic floor muscles to prevent **and** cure incontinence.

**Learn more and get bonus material at
www.innerbalancept.com.**

Resources For Incontinence

National Association for Continence (NAFC)
P.O. Box 1019
Charleston, SC 29402-1019
1.800.BLADDER
www.nafc.org

The Simon Foundation for Continence
P.O. Box 815
Wilmette, IL 60091
1.800.23Simon
www.simonfoundation.org

American Urogynecology Society
2025 M Street NW, Suite 800
Washington, DC 20036
1.202.367.1167
www.augs.org

Section on Women's Health
American Physical Therapy Association
8400 Westpark Drive, 2nd Floor
McClean, VA 22102
1.703.610.0224
www.womenshealthapta.org

National Kidney and Urologic Diseases Information Clearinghouse
3 Information Way
Bethesda, MD 20892-3580
1.800.891.5390
www.kidney.niddk.nih.gov

Glossary

Abdominal cavity–the part of the body containing the digestive organs and bounded by the diaphragm and the pelvis; the belly

Abscess–a swollen area within body tissue, containing an accumulation of pus

Anterior pelvic tilt–when the position of the pelvis is tilted forward toward the toes

Autonomic nervous system (ANS)–the part of the nervous system responsible for control of the bodily functions not consciously directed, such as breathing, the heartbeat, and digestive processes; has a sympathetic and parasympathetic division

Bladder–a distensible membranous sac that serves for the temporary retention of the urine; situated in the pelvis in front of the rectum, it receives the urine from the two ureters and discharges it at intervals into the urethra through an orifice closed by a sphincter

Bladder irritation–the stimulation of the bladder to produce an active response

Bladder opening–the aperture or gap allowing access to the bladder

Bladder spasm–a sudden involuntary muscular contraction or convulsive movement in the bladder

Body mechanics–exercises designed to improve posture, coordination, and stamina during correct body movements

Bowels–the part of the alimentary canal below the stomach; the intestine

Caffeine–a crystalline compound that is found especially in tea and coffee plants and is a stimulant of the central nervous system

Central nervous system–the complex of nerve tissues that controls the activities of the body; comprises the brain and spinal cord

Colonic inertia – the abnormal passage of waste through the digestive system where the function of the digestive system may be impaired

Comprehensive home program–a complete program designed to be completed at home

Concentrated urine–urine that is present in a high proportion relative to other substances; having had water, or other diluting agent, removed or reduced

Consistent rate of fill–the unchanging speed with which something moves, happens, or changes; concerning the bladder, the unchanging speed with which it fills with urine

Constipation–a condition in which there is difficulty in emptying the bowels, usually associated with hardened feces

Cystoscopic procedure–the insertion of an instrument into the urethra for examining the urinary bladder

Diaphragm–a dome-shaped, muscular partition separating the thorax from the abdomen in mammals; plays a major role in breathing, as its contraction increases the volume of the thorax, and so inflates the lungs

Dilute–make (a liquid) thinner or weaker by adding water or another solvent to it

Distraction–a thing that prevents someone from giving full attention to something else

Exhale–breathe out in a deliberate manner

FAQs–frequently asked questions

Fight or flight response–the instinctive physiological response to a threatening situation, which readies one either to resist forcibly or to run away

Good fluid–a drink that does not irritate the bladder

Gravity–the force that attracts a body toward the center of the earth, or toward any other physical body having mass

Intermittent catheterization – insertion of a catheter into a patient or body cavity, like the bladder, at irregular intervals

Internal pelvic organs–body organs that lie inside the pelvis, like the bladder, uterus, and ovaries

Invisible irritant–good fluids that would otherwise keep the bladder calm but that are not being regularly consumed; as a result, the bladder becomes irritated

Involuntary muscle contraction–the process by which a muscle becomes or is made shorter and tighter without will or conscious control

Kegel–an exercise to strengthen the pelvic floor muscles, in which the levator muscles are squeezed and then released for a number of repetitions; they are used to treat urinary incontinence, or to prepare for or recover from childbirth

Miralax–a medicine given to stimulate or facilitate evacuation of the bowels

Muscle–a band or bundle of fibrous tissue in a human or animal body that has the ability to contract, producing movement in or maintaining the position of parts of the body

Neutral bladder environment–urine that is neither acidic nor alkaline, thereby keeping the bladder calm

Organ prolapse–a slipping forward or down of one of the organs of the body; for example, a prolapsed bladder, uterus, or rectum

Overactive bladder–excessively or abnormally active (or contracting) bladder

Panicked state–a sudden uncontrollable fear or anxiety, often causing wildly unthinking behavior; often the result of an urgent bladder signal

Pelvic brace–an exercise that combines a pelvic floor (Kegel) contraction with a transverse abdominal contraction

Pelvic floor dysfunction–abnormality or impairment in the function of the pelvic floor (Kegel) muscles

Pelvis–the large bony structure near the base of the spine to which the hind limbs or legs are attached in humans and many other vertebrates

Peristalsis–the involuntary constriction and relaxation of the muscles of the intestine or another canal, creating wave like movements that push the contents of the canal forward

Physical therapy–the treatment of disease, injury, or deformity by physical methods such as massage, heat treatment, manual techniques and exercise rather than by drugs or surgery

Posterior pelvic tilt–when the position of the pelvis is tilted backward toward the head

Posture–the position of a person's body when standing or sitting; good posture places the muscles surrounding the pelvis in the best possible position to maximize the strengthening process

Precautions–measures taken to prevent something dangerous, unpleasant, or inconvenient from happening

Bladder relaxation–the loss of tension in the bladder when it ceases to contract

Roll-In–an exercise performed by rolling the knees into each other to elicit a pelvic floor (Kegel) contraction

Roll-Out–an exercise performed by rolling the knees out and away from each other to elicit a pelvic floor (Kegel) contraction

Strain–a force tending to pull or stretch something to an extreme or damaging degree; for example, to strain with urination or defecation

Thirst–a feeling of needing or wanting to drink something

Transverse abdominal contraction–an exercise performed to elicit a contraction of the transverse abdominal muscles

Urge–a strong desire or impulse

Urinary frequency–the need to urinate more often than considered normal; to urinate greater than 4-6 times in 24 hours

Urinary incontinence–unintentional loss of urine

Urinary tract–the series of channels by which the urine passes from the renal pelvis out of the body

Urinary urgency–a sudden need to urinate requiring immediate action or attention

Urine–a watery, typically yellowish fluid stored in the bladder and discharged through the urethra; one of the body's chief means of eliminating excess water and salt; also contains nitrogen compounds such as urea and other waste substances removed from the blood by the kidneys

Urodynamic testing - the diagnostic study of pressure in the bladder, in treating incontinence

Urologist–a doctor who specializes in the function and disorders of the urinary system

Voluntary muscle contraction–the process in which a muscle becomes or is made shorter and tighter with free will or conscious control

For More Information
On This Topic And Others
See My Social Media Sites Below

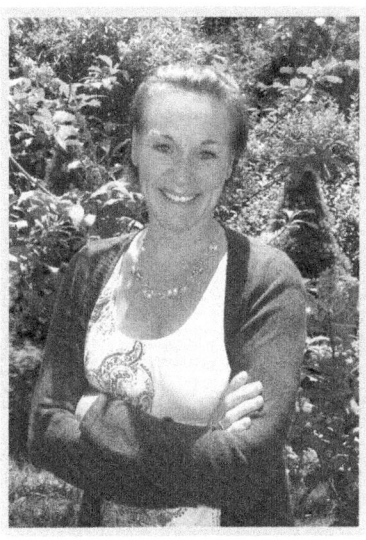

Leslie M. Parker, MPT, CDT
Inner Balance Physical Therapy
43 Harold L. Dow Highway, Unit 4
Eliot, Maine 03903
Phone: 207.703.0255 Fax: 603.617.2665

Website: www.innerbalancept.com

Facebook: www.facebook.com/InnerBalancePhysicalTherapy

Twitter: www.twitter.com/ppods6511

Pinterest: www.pinterest.com/ppods651

Instagram: ppods651

Made in the USA
Coppell, TX
03 November 2020